Cor

Dropping Acid
Reflux Diet
Cookbook.

Easy Anti Acid

Diet Meal Plans & Recipes

to Heal GERD and LPR.

Causes for Acid Reflux.

Contents

Chapter 1. Understanding Acid Reflux and GERD

Acid Alkaline Balance for good Health and Diet

The modern day diet we are consuming is way more acidic than it previously was. This imbalanced acid alkali diet is the reason for very serious and chronic medical complications like arthritis and osteoporosis. Creating a balanced acid alkali diet plan is very critical for having access to a healthy lifestyle, and it is very easy to achieve.

Apart from weight loss, the alkaline diet is high in energy; lowers the risk of having kidney complications, type-2 diabetes and various other diseases like lactic-acid build up (aka leg cramps); reduces joint pain, and improves both your skin and bone health.

History

According to the research of R. Curtis Morris, the Stone Age diet was highly alkaline in nature, and that has been altered considerably to highly acidic in nature to the present day. This has been the reason for serious medical complications, as our diets have posed to be more acidic while our bodies are designed to have a balanced alkaline diet for effective and healthy working.

Importance

According to the research of Dr. L. Frassetto, any diet which is more inclined towards acid-creating foods and reluctant in creating alkaline-creating foods, including include bicarbonates and potassium in particular, results in a low grade form of acidity in the body.

There are numerous health-related complications which are credited towards an imbalance in the acid-alkali diet. As per Regina Cseuz, acidity is strongly linked to having rheumatoid arthritis and can pose to be fatal. Dr. David Bushinsky has argued and presented his finding of the association between osteoporosis and acidity which indeed is a result of imbalanced acid alkali content of the diet.

Sources of Acids

Dr. Friedrich Manz and Dr. Thomas Remer calculated the acidic and alkaline nature of many foods in 1995. They measured the PRAL (aka potential renal acid load) per 3.5 oz. of every substance. They defined a negative value to be more alkaline and vice versa.

Cheese has the highest average PRAL of +23.6 posing to be very highly acidic. Milk has +0.7 (considerably neutral), and meat has an average PRAL of +9.5.

Sources of Alkaline

Veggies and fruits are known to be highly alkaline in nature. The PRAL of spinach and fresh carrots and celery have their respective PRALs to be -14.0, -4.9 and -5.2. The PRAL of raisins is known to be -21.0, while fruits like apricot, black currents, and bananas have an average PRAL ranging from -5 to -6.

Balancing the Diet

It is understood that meats and grains are acidic in nature while veggies and fruits are alkaline in nature. To balance your diet, simply balance the PRAL values of both the categories. If you have 3 oz. of meat having PRAL +9.5, you need either 3 oz. of spinach or 7 oz. carrots to achieve -9.5 PRAL to make your diet acid alkali balanced.

What causes acid reflux?

There are various reasons for a higher risk of having acid reflux disease. Some of them are as follows:

1. Stomach Complications

A hiatal hernia is generally considered one of the most common reasons for acid reflux, and surprisingly, it can happen to anybody regardless of age. It is due to the movement of the lower esophageal sphincter (LES) and the upper portion of the stomach over the diaphragm. The diaphragm basically protects your esophagus from acid, but in the case of a hiatal hernia, it reaches the esophagus.

2. Pregnancy

Acid reflux can be observed in women during their first pregnancy due to the increased pressure from the gradually growing fetus in addition to enhanced levels of hormones. It is at its peak in the 3rd trimester, and the symptoms of acid reflux start fading away as soon after delivery.

3. Smoking

Apart from increasing the danger of esophagus cancer, following harms of smoking are considered to be responsible for causing acid reflux:

- Enhancement of Acid Secretion
- Reduced Muscle Function of LES
- Reduced Production of Saliva. (Saliva is effective in acid neutralization)
- Damaged Membranes of Mucus
- Impaired Reflexes of Throat Muscles

4. Diet

Lying in bed immediately after consuming food or having a larger meal can result in initiating heartburning and various other symptoms of acid reflux, i.e. problems in food swallowing, dry cough, etc. Following daily used foods are known to be causing acid reflux:

- Carbonated drinks
- Alcohol
- Spicy foods, i.e. including chilies and curries.
- Chocolate
- Tea or Coffee including both decaffeinated or regular.
- Citrus fruits, i.e. lemons or oranges etc.
- Fried or Fatty foods
- Onions and Garlic
- Tomato containing foods, i.e. pizza, salsa or spaghetti sauce
- Mint

There are many other reasons for acid reflux that are:
- Obesity and Overweightness
- Eating right before sleeping
- Consuming larger meals and afterward either bending over the waist or lying in the bed
- Consuming muscle relaxants, various BP controlling medications, and even aspirin or ibuprofen, etc.

Dietary Acid Damage: Why It should be feared?

People having chronic kidney conditions may be exposed to a higher risk of kidney failure if their diet is high in acidic content. According to JASN, kidney patients should consume more fruits and veggies and reduce the consumption of meats to keep their kidneys in shape and healthy. A person's nutrition is the definition of his health, and it can be very critical to remain healthy. A healthy diet provides access to a healthy lifestyle, and any abruptions in healthy diets can lead to serious medical complications. The consumption of higher acidic diets can result in serious diseases including kidney failures and related complications. Highly acidic diets include meats, while lower acidic diets include fruits.

Acid Reflex, Esophagus, and Cancer

The esophagus is a closed passage which connects the throat to the stomach and passes the food from the mouth to the guts for digestion. Acid reflux can cause esophagus cancer, and this cancer can even spread off to various other parts of the body and that is called metastasis. Initially, the esophagus cancer starts in the inner layer of the esophagus and gradually transfers to the other layers before further transmission.

There are basically two types of esophagus cancer, i.e., squamous cell carcinoma while the other is known as adenocarcinoma. Adenocarcinoma is formed due to gland cells. It is caused by the replacement of squamous cells by gland cells in the esophagus. This usually happens in the lower portion of the esophagus which is nearer to the stomach and is credited to the high rate of exposure to acid to the lower esophagus.

Acid Reflux and Weight Gain

According to a published report in a journal known as the New England Journal of Medicine, gastroesophageal flux disease (GERD) is known to be directly connected to weight gaining even in small proportions. Researchers have also argued that it is associated with little weight gains without the individual being overweight at all.

You can be more exposed to the risk of having GERD if you have put on excess weight or even so little that you can't be classified as overweight. According to Dr. B. Jacobson who is a study author at the Boston University School of Medicine, any form of excessive weight negatively impacts your health. If anybody who has normal weight puts on extra weight, no matter how small, can be more likely to be exposed to the risk of having GERD.

Effects of Acid Alkaline Imbalance

A balanced acid alkali diet is the critically important factor towards attaining a healthy and nutritious lifestyle. Any imbalance in acid alkali content of your diet can result in medical complications which can be at some point very seriously.

Dr. William Howard Hay in his book called 'A New Health Era' which was published in 1933 pondered hat the root cause of all the diseases was due to autotoxication which occurs due to the accumulation of acid inside the body. Since then many nutritionists, herbalists, doctors, etc. have supported this theory and argued that any imbalance in acid alkali content of your diet causes serious health problems and creates a weaker immune system which furthermore paves the way for disease to   grow   inside   your   body.

It is also known that opting for a balanced diet on the pH scale provides your body with effective energy, nutrition, and safety while allowing the smooth and healthy functioning of your body to curb and resist any disease.

Testing for pH Balance

By reading so much about acid-alkali balance, you must be inquisitive about how to check the equilibrium between both of them. As tricky as it sounds, it is very easy instead. Simply go to a medical store or any online retailer and ask for pH test strips.

You can conduct a pH test whenever you want, but it is preferred to undergo this test in the mornings. The reason is that in the mornings your body tends to be more acidic in nature and this acidity increases the early you measure it. The aim is simply to have your urine pH levels ranging somewhere between 6.5 to 7.5 while keeping in view hat these levels may significantly vary.

In case of saliva, your pH result should be as same as your urine. For saliva pH testing, wait approximately 2 hours after eating your food and then measure it. Fill your mouth with saliva and then take a gulp unless you are sure that your saliva is completely clean now. Afterward, simply place some of your salivae on top of the pH scale, and it will give you the results.

It is considered to be fine if you cannot alter your diet completely in accordance to the acid-alkali balancing. You can also aim to have a 70% to 30% ratio of alkaline to acidic foods. Apart from your diet, stress levels are also known for affecting your body pH levels. To avoid getting stressed out, enhance your water consumptions, eat loads of veggies and practice deep breathing effectively to lower down the acidic levels of your body.

Chapter 2. Relationship Between Food & Symptoms

Understanding the Role of protein, Carbohydrates, and Fats in Healing Dietary Acid Damage

A combination of lean proteins, comparatively slow low-carbs, and fats can prove to be very pivotal to lose weight which indeed helps in lowering the risk of having GERD in the first place. Beginners should go for a protein shake in breakfast for having an effective and faster approach towards weight loss.

Lowering the intake of foods having higher sugar impact can reduce the risk of GERD. Research also concluded that simple carbs could be more contributing to GERD as compared to dietary fats.

Digestive enzymes can be consumed so that fats and proteins are broken down and digested more conveniently in the stomach and thus the symptoms like bloating gas are less likely to happen.

Acidity and Alkalinity

On a pH scale, zero is considered to be acidic while 14 is considered to be entirely alkaline. The pH 7 is considered to be neutral. These pH levels actually vary through our bodies. The pH of our blood is ranging between 7.35 to 7.45 and is considered to be slightly alkaline in nature. The alkaline diet is very effective in keeping your blood pH levels maintained.

Breaking Acid-Generation Habits and Establishing Acid-Reduction Practices:

1. Eat Green

Alkaline foods like legumes, fruits, roots, nuts, and veggies should be consumed in abundance. Opt for these foods rather than meats and grains. Go for green or dark veggies like avocados, beetroot, kale, spinach, etc.

2. Lower Acidic Foods

It's not necessary to completely boycott meats, refined sugars, dairy, and grains, but it is preferred to lower their intake to lower down the acidity of your body.

3. Reduce Alcohol Consumption

Alcoholic drinks are known to be high in sugar and extremely acidic in nature. They are not meant to be removed entirely, but their intake should be lowered down considerably.

4. Drink Alkaline Water:

Water is very vital for our health. It is essential to consume 8 to 10 glasses of alkaline water daily to have access to a healthy lifestyle. Instead of tap water (pH 6.5 to 7), opt for alkaline water (pH 9) to effectively balance acid-alkaline levels in the body. Its molecules are small and can permeate your body easily, keeping you hydrated for a long time.

5. Opt Natural Energy Boosting Beverages:
Say no to caffeine and sugar-based drinks. Go for natural alkaline drinks like lemon water, peppermint tea, etc. which are known to clean the digestive system, strengthen the metabolism, and balance out the acidity of the body.

6. Exercise Properly:
Effectively exercise 30 minutes every day to counter acidity. The sweat provides a different medium for the acidity to leave while helping the blood getting alkalize and oxygenate.

7. Avoid Stress
Stress is known for generating high acid levels in the body so try avoiding it by practicing deep breaths, yoga or long walks, etc.

Food Allergies, Sensitivities and Intolerance
The difference between food allergy and food intolerance needs to be understood comprehensively.
Actual food allergy is very rare as compared to intolerance. Approximately 8% of children while 4% of adults are affected

by it. It is basically a quick reaction by the immune system to proteins in some foods, i.e. nuts and milk, and can be easily verified by a test conducted in a lab. While on the other hand food intolerance is a common reaction and a delayed response to some natural or artificial chemicals in foods involving various foods. There is no certain laboratory oriented test for this, so it is tested by removing a diet with various challenges.

Understand your reaction and preferences to food while turning towards the acid reflux diet plan and note the reactions of your body to the meal you are consuming for effective working of the plan. There are mainly five versatile categories for food intolerance symptoms, and every family member can be having any of them. These include:

- Asthma, running nose, nose, and ear infections
- Moth ulcers, stomach aches, constipation, urinary urgency diarrhea, etc.
- Eczema, skin rashes, hives, etc.
- Headaches or migraines
- Depression, anxiety, restlessness, etc.

Chapter-3. Creating Acid-Alkaline Balance:

1. Eat Small Meals

Eat small and nutritious. Maintain a ratio of 70-30 percent alkaline to acidic foods.

2. Stop Eating at Least Four Hours Before Bedtime

Posture plays an important role in having the risk of GERD. Always eat 3-4 hours prior to sleeping to avoid acid reflux.

3. Wear Loose Clothing

Lose clothing lets your abdomen relax, and there is no pressure on it. This can lower down your acid reflux and can be very effective for overweight people.

4. If You are Overweight, Lose Weight

An increase in weight no matter how tiny the increment is, means a higher risk of having GERD. Exercise properly to lose weight effectively.

5. Minimize Fat in Foods

Always go for low-fat foods to avoid the risk of GERD. Food categories are further explained in the next chapter.

6. Avoid Foods That May Increase IAP

IAP is a result bacterial overgrowth, and mal digested carbs. Increased IAP results in GERD. It is recommended to avoid any foods which are known to be causing IAP.

7. Avoid Foods or Substances That Weaken Your LES

There are numerous causes for the weakening of lower esophageal sphincter, and almost all of them can be easily avoided. Following are some of them.

8. Overeating or Being Overweight

Overeating or overweightness leads to excessive pressure build-up on the LES as the stomach swells. After some time, the LES loses its durability and shape and thus starts allowing acid to reach upwards which furthers weakens it.

9. Smoking

The chemicals and toxins found in cigarette smoke make the membranes of the LES weak, it also increases the acidity levels of the stomach thus affecting the LES more than normal stomach fluids do.

10. Alcohol Consumption

Alcohol is known to make the LES weak, and it lowers its ability to close. It allows acid to flow up the LES by relaxing the muscles and thus damages it.

11. Various Medications

Medicines like BP meds, sleeping pills, antibiotics, etc. are known to keep the muscles of LES relaxed causing the acid to flow upward and damaging it critically.

12. Certain Foods

Trigger foods are not recommended for people with GERD. High-fat foods also relax the LES muscles and cause it damage.

Chapter-4 Food Tables.

Foods Not to Eat:

The following foods are known to make GERD worse and tend to be acidic in nature. Their intake should be lowered and reduced very much.

- Foods which have high fats and oil (these foods may result in the relaxation of the sphincter in the stomach)
- Meats (it is highly acidic in nature while having a higher amount of fatty acids and cholesterol levels)
- Foods which are the sources of saturated fats. These include cheese (highly acidic in nature) and milk
- Excessive amounts of salts
- Mint
- Chocolate
- Carbonated beverages (sodas)
- Caffeine
- Acidic drinks which include coffee and orange juice etc.
- Acidic foods which consist of tomato sauce etc.

Foods to Eat:

The following foods are known to be alkaline in nature and can be used to avoid the risk of having GERD. These foods should be consumed in abundance.

- Carbs present in various veggies, fruits, and certain whole grains

- Proteins from trout, lentils, lean poultry, salmon, and beans which are low in cholesterol levels.
- Foods rich in vitamin C content, e.g. veggies and fruits
- Green veggies like spinach, asparagus, Brussels sprouts, broccoli, and kale, etc.
- High fibered food especially high in soluble fiber foods is known to lower down the risk of GERD.
- Highly fibered (rich in potassium and magnesium) fruits like apples, melons, avocados, bananas, peaches, pears, and berries, etc.
- Eggs (irrespective of their cholesterol levels)
- Avoid foods or substances that increase acidity
- Straightforwardly lower the intake of acidic foods like meat and grains etc.
- Eat more alkaline foods
- Consume more veggies and fruits like broccoli, spinach, bananas, etc.

Chapter-5. FDA's pH Food List

Item	Approximate pH
Abalone	6.10 - 6.50
Abalone mushroom	5.0
Ackees	5.50
Aloe vera	6.10
Aloe Juice	6.00 - 6.80
Anchovies	6.50
Anchovies, stuffed w/capers, in olive oil	5.58
Antipasto	5.60
Apple, baked with sugar	3.20 - 3.55
Apple, eating	3.30 - 4.00
Apple Delicious	3.90
Golden Delicious	3.60
Jonathan	3.33
McIntosh	3.34
Juice	3.35 - 4.00
Sauce	3.10 - 3.60
Winesap	3.47
Apricots	3.30 - 4.80
Canned	3.40 - 3.78
Dried, stewed	3.30 - 3.51

Nectar	3.78
Pureed	3.42 - 3.83
Strained	3.72 - 3.95
Arrowroot Crackers	6.63 - 6.80
Arrowroot Cruel	6.37 - 6.87
Artichokes	5.50 - 6.00
Artichokes, canned, acidified	4.30 - 4.60
Artichokes, French, cooked	5.60 - 6.00
Artichokes, Jerusalem, cooked	5.93 - 6.00
Asparagus	6.00 - 6.70
Buds	6.70
Stalks	6.10
Asparagus, cooked	6.03 - 6.16
Asparagus, canned	5.00 - 6.00
Asparagus, frozen, cooked	6.35 - 6.48
Asparagus, green, canned	5.20 - 5.32
Asparagus, strained	4.80 - 5.09
Avocados	6.27 - 6.58
Baby corn	5.20
Baby Food Soup, unstrained	5.95 - 6.05
Bamboo Shoots	5.10 - 6.20
Bamboo Shoots, preserved	3.50 - 4.60
Bananas	4.50 - 5.20
Bananas, red	4.58 - 4.75
Banana, yellow	5.00 - 5.29

Barley, cooked	5.19 - 5.32
Basil pesto	4.90
Bass, sea, broiled	6.58 - 6.78
Bass, striped, broiled	6.50 - 6.70
Beans	5.60 - 6.50
Black	5.78 - 6.02
Boston style	5.05 - 5.42
Kidney	5.40 - 6.00
Lima	6.50
Soy	6.00 - 6.60
String	5.60
Wax	5.30 - 5.70
Beans, pork & tomato sauce, canned	5.10 - 5.80
Beans, refried	5.90
Beans, vegetarian, tomato sauce, canned	5.32
Beets	5.30 - 6.60
Beets, cooked	5.23 - 6.50
Beets, canned, acidified	4.30 - 4.60
Beets, canned	4.90 - 5.80
Beets, chopped	5.32 - 5.56
Beets, strained	5.32 - 5.56
Bird's nest soup	7.20 - 7.60
Blackberries, Washington	3.85 - 4.50

Blueberries, Maine	3.12 - 3.33
Blueberries, frozen	3.11 - 3.22
Bluefish, Boston, filet, broiled	6.09 - 6.50
Bran Flakes	5.45 - 5.67
All Bran	5.59 - 6.19
Bread, white	5.00 - 6.20
Bread, Boston, brown	6.53
Bread, Cracked wheat	5.43 - 5.50
Bread, pumpernickel	5.40
Bread, Rye	5.20 - 5.90
Bread, whole wheat	5.47 - 5.85
Breadfruit, cooked	5.33
Broccoli, cooked	6.30 - 6.52
Broccoli, frozen, cooked	6.30 - 6.85
Broccoli, canned	5.20 - 6.00
Brussels sprout	6.00 - 6.30
Buttermilk	4.41 - 4.83
Cabbage	5.20 - 6.80
Green	5.50 - 6.75
Red	5.60 - 6.00
Savoy	6.30
White	6.20
Cactus	4.70
Calamari (Squid)	5.80
Cantaloupe	6.13 - 6.58

Capers	6.00
Carp	6.00
Carrots	5.88 - 6.40
Carrots, canned	5.18 - 5.22
Carrots, chopped	5.30 - 5.56
Carrots, cooked	5.58 - 6.03
Carrots, pureed	4.55 - 5.80
Carrots, strained	5.10 - 5.10
Cauliflower	5.60
Cauliflower, cooked	6.45 - 6.80
Caviar, American	5.70 - 6.00
Celery	5.70 - 6.00
Celery, cooked	5.37 - 5.92
Celery Knob, cooked	5.71 - 5.85
Cereal, strained	6.44 - 6.45
Chayote (mirliton), cooked	6.00 - 6.30
Cheese, American, mild	4.98
Cheese, Camembert	7.44
Cheese, Cheddar	5.90
Cheese, Cottage	4.75 - 5.02
Cheese, Cream, Philadelphia	4.10 - 4.79
Cheese Dip	5.80
Cheese, Edem	5.40
Cheese, Old English	6.15
Cheese, Roquefort	5.10 - 5.98

Cheese, Parmesan	5.20 - 5.30
Cheese, Snippy	5.18 - 5.2l
Cheese, Stilton	5.70
Cheese, Swiss Gruyere	5.68 - 6.62
Cherries, California	44.01 -.54
Cherries, frozen	3.32 - 3.37
Cherries, black, canned	3.82 - 3.93
Cherries, Maraschino	3.47 - 3.52
Cherries, red, Water pack	3.25 - 3.82
Cherries, Royal Ann	3.80 - 3.83
Chicory	5.90 - 6.05
Chili Sauce, acidified	2.77 - 3.70
Chives	5.20 - 6.31
Clams	6.00 - 7.1
Clam Chowder, New England	6.40
Coconut, fresh	5.50 - 7.80
Coconut milk	6.10 - 7.00
Coconut preserves	3.80 - 7.00
Codfish, boiled	5.30 - 6.10
Cod Liver	6.20
Conch	7.52 - 8.40
Congee	6.40
Corn	5.90 - 7.30
Corn, canned	5.90- 6.50
Corn Flakes	4.90 - 5.38

Corn, frozen, cooked	7.33 - 7.68
Corn, Golden Bantam, cooked on the cob	6.22 - 7.04
Crab Meat	6.50 - 7.00
Crabapple Jelly, corn	2.93 - 3.02
Cranberry Juice, canned	2.30 - 2.52
Crabmeat, cooked	6.62 - 6.98
Cream, 20 percent	6.50 - 6.68
Cream, 40 percent	6.44 - 6.80
Cream of Asparagus	6.10
Cream of Coconut, canned	5.51 - 5.87
Cream of Potato soup	6.00
Cream of Wheat, cooked	6.06 - 6.16
Chrysanthemum drink	6.50
Cucumbers	5.12 - 5.78
Cucumbers, Dill pickles	3.20 - 3.70
Cucumbers, pickled	4.20 - 4.60
Curry sauce	6.00
Curry Paste,acidified	4.60 - 4.80
Cuttlefish	6.30
Dates, canned	6.20 - 6.40
Dates, Dromedary	4.14 - 4.88
Dungeness Crab Meat Eggplant	5.50 - 6.50
Eggs, new-laid, whole	6.58
White	7.96

Yolk	6.10
Eel	6.20
Escarole	5.70 - 6.00
Enchilada sauce	4.40 - 4.70
Fennel (Anise)	5.48 - 5.88
Fennel, cooked	5.80 - 6.02
Figs, Calamyrna	5.05 - 5.98
Figs, canned	4.92 - 5.00
Flounder, boiled	6.10 - 6.90
Flounder, fi1et, broiled	6.39 - 6.89
Four bean salad	5.60
Fruit cocktail	3.60 - 4.00
Garlic	5.80
Gelatin Dessert	2.60
Gelatin, plain jell	6.08
Gherkin Ginger	5.60 - 5.90
Ginseng , Korean drink	6.00 - 6.50
Gooseberries	2.80 - 3.10
Graham Crackers	7.10 - 7.92
Grapes, canned	3.50 - 4.50
Grapes, Concord	2.80 - 3.00
Grapes, Lady Finger	3.51 - 3.58
Grapes, Malaga	3.71 - 3.78
Grapes, Niagara	2.80 - 3.27
Grapes, Ribier	3.70 - 3.80

Grapes, Seedless	2.90 - 3.82
Grapes, Tokyo	3.50 - 3.84
Grapefruit	3.00 - 3.75
Grapefruit, canned	3.08 - 3.32
Grapefruit Juice, canned	2.90 - 3.25
Grass jelly	5.80 - 7.20
Greens, Mixed, chopped	5.05 - 5.22
Greens, Mixed, strained	5.22 - 5.30
Grenadine Syrup	2.31
Guava nectar	5.50
Guava, canned	3.37 - 4. 10
Guava Jelly	3.73
Haddock, Filet, broiled	6.17 - 6.82
Hearts of Palm	5.70
Herring	6.10
Hominy, cooked	6.00 - 7.50
Honey	3.70 - 4.20
Honey Aloe	4.70
Horseradish, freshly ground	5.35
Huckleberries, cooked with sugar	3.38 - 3.43
Jackfruit	4.80 - 6.80
Jam, fruit	3.50 - 4.50
Jellies, fruit	3.00 - 3.50
Jujube	5.20

Junket type Dessert:	
Raspberry	6.27
Vanilla	6.49
Kale, cooked	6.36 - 6.80
Ketchup	3.89 - 3.92
Kippered, Herring, Marshall	5.75 - 6.20
Herring, Pickled	4.50 - 5.00
Kelp	6.30
Kumquat, Florida	3.64 - 4.25
Leeks	5.50 - 6.17
Leeks, cooked	5.49 - 6.10
Lemon Juice	2.00 - 2.60
Lentils, cooked	6.30 - 6.83
Lentil Soup	5.80
Lettuce	5.80 - 6.15
Lettuce, Boston	5.89 - 6.05
Lettuce, Iceberg	5.70 - 6.13
Lime	2.00 - 2.80
Lobster bisque	6.90
Lobster soup	5.70
Lobster, cooked	7.10 - 7.43
Loganberries	2.70 - 3.50
Loquat (Maybe acidified to pH 3.8)	5.10
Lotus Root	6.90

Lychee	4.70 - 5.01
Macaroni, cooked	5.10 - 6.41
Mackerel, King, boiled	6.26 - 6.50
Mackerel, Spanish, broiled	6.07 - 6.36
Mackerel, canned	5.90 - 6.40
Mangoes, ripe	3.40 - 4.80
Mangoes, green	5.80 - 6.00
Mangosteen ?	4.50 -5.00
Maple syrup	5.15
Maple syrup, light (Acidified)	4.60
Matzos	5.70
Mayhaw (a variety of strawberry)	3.27 - 3.86
Melba Toast	5.08 - 5.30
Melon, Casaba	5.78 - 6.00
Melons, Honeydew	6.00 - 6.67
Melons, Persian	5.90 - 6.38
Milk, cow	6.40 - 6.80
Milk, Acidophilus	4.09 - 4.25
Milk, condensed	6.33
Milk evaporated	5.90 - 6.30

Milk, Goat's	6.48
Milk, peptonized	7.10
Milk, Sour, fine curd	4.70 - 5.65
Milkfish	5.30
Mint Jelly	3.01
Molasses	4.90 - 5.40
Muscadine (A variety of grape)	3.20 - 3.40
Mushrooms	6.00 - 6.70
Mushrooms, cooked	6.00 - 6.22
Mushroom Soup, Cream of, canned	5.95 - 6.40
Mussels	6.00 - 6.85
Mustard	3.55 - 6.00
Nata De Coco	5.00
Nectarines	3.92 - 4.18
Noodles, boiled	6.08 - 6.50
Oatmeal, cooked	6.20 - 6.60
Octopus	6.00 - 6.50
Okra, cooked	5.50 - 6.60
Olives, black	6.00 - 7.00
Olives, green, fermented	3.60 - 4.60
Olives, ripe	6.00 -7.50
Onions, pickled	3.70 - 4.60
Onions, red	5.30 - 5.80
Onion white	5.37 - 5.85
Onions, yellow	5.32 - 5.60

Oranges, Florida	3.69 - 4.34
Oranges, Florida "color added."	3.60 - 3.90
Orange Juice, California	3.30 - 4.19
Orange, Juice Florida	3.30 - 4.15
Orange, Marmalade	3.00 - 3.33
Oysters	5.68 - 6.17
Oyster, smoked	6.00
Oyster mushrooms	5.00 - 6.00
Palm, the heart of	6.70
Papaya	5.20 - 6.00
Papaya Marmalade	3.53 - 4.00
Parsley	5.70 - 6.00
Parsnip	5.30 - 5.70
Parsnips, cooked	5.45 - 5.65
Pate	5.90
Peaches	3.30 - 4.05
Peaches, canned	3.70 - 4.20
Peaches, cooked with sugar	3.55 -3.72
Peaches, frozen	3.28 - 3.35
Peanut Butter	6.28
Peanut Soup	7.5
Pears, Bartlett	3.50 - 4.60
Pears, canned	4.00 - 4.07
Pears, Sickle cooked w/sugar	4.04 - 4.21
Pear Nectar	4.03

Peas, canned	5.70 - 6.00
Peas, Chick, Garbanzo	6.48 - 6.80
Peas, cooked	6.22 - 6.88
Peas, dried (split green), cooked	6.45 - 6.80
Peas, dried (split yellow), cooked	6.43 - 6.62
Peas, frozen, cooked	6.40 - 6.70
Peas, pureed	4.90 - 5.85
Pea Soup, Cream of, Canned	5.70
Peas, strained	5.91 - 6.12
Peppers	4.65 - 5.45
Peppers, green	5.20 - 5.93
Persimmons	4.42 - 4.70
Pickles, fresh pack	5.10 - 5.40
Pimiento	4.40 - 4.90
Pimento, canned, acidified	4.40 - 4.60
Pineapple	3.20 - 4.00
Pineapple, canned	3.35 - 4.10
Pineapple Juice, canned	3.30 - 3.60
Plum Nectar	3.45
Plums, Blue	2.80 - 3.40
Plums, Damson	2.90 - 3.10
Plums, Frozen	3.22 - 3.42
Plums, Green Gage	3.60 - 4.30
Plums, Green Gage, canned	3.22 - 3.32
Plums, Red	3.60 - 4.30

Plums, spiced	3.64
Plums, Yellow	3.90 - 4.45
Pollack, filet, broiled	6.72 - 6.82
Pomegranate	2.93 - 3.20
Porgy, broiled	6.40 - 6.49
Pork & Beans, rts.	5.70
Potatoes	5.40 - 5.90
Mashed	5.10
Prunes, dried, stewed	3.63 - 3.92
Sweet	5.30 - 5.60
Tubers	5.70
Potato Soup	5.90
Prune Juice	3.95 - 3.97
Prune, pureed	3.60 - 4.30
Prune, strained	3.58 - 3.83
Puffed Rice	6.27 - 6.40
Puffed Wheat	5.26 - 5.77
Pumpkin	4.90 - 5.50
Quince, fresh, stewed	3.12 - 3.40
Quince Jelly	3.70
Radishes, red	5.85 - 6.05
Radishes, white	5.52 - 5.69
Raisins, seedless	3.80 - 4.10
Rambutan (Thailand)	4.90
Raspberries	3.22 - 3.95

Raspberries, frozen	3.18 - 3.26
Raspberries, New Jersey	3.50 - 3.82
Raspberry Jam	2.87 - 3.17
Razor Clams	6.20
Razor shell (sea asparagus)	6.00
Rattan, Thailand	5.20
Red Ginseng	5.50
Red Pepper Relish	3.10 - 3.62
Rhubarb, California, stewed	3.20 - 3.34
Rhubarb	3.10 - 3.40
Canned	3.40
Rice (all cooked)	
Brown	6.20 - 6.80
Krispies	5.40 - 5.73
White	6.00 - 6.70
Wild	6.00 - 6.50
Rolls, white	5.46 - 5.52
Romaine	5.78 - 6.06
Salmon, fresh, boiled	5.85 - 6.50
Salmon, fresh, broiled	5.36 - 6.40
Salmon, Red Alaska, canned	6.07 - 6.16
Salsa Sardines	5.70 - 6.60
Sardine, Portuguese, in olive oil	5.42 - 5.93
Satay sauce	5.00
Sauce, Enchilada	5.50

Sauce, Fish	4.93 - 5.02
Sauce, Shrimp	7.01 - 7.27
Sauerkraut	3.30 - 3.60
Scallion	6.20
Scallop	6.00
Scotch Broth.	5.92
Sea Snail (Top shell)	6.00
Shad Roe, sauteed	5.70 - 5.90
Shallots, cooked	5.30 - 5.70
Sherbet, raspberry	3.69
Sherry-wine	3.37
Shredded Ralston	5.32 - 5.60
Shredded Wheat	6.05 - 6.49
Shrimp	6.50 - 7.00
Shrimp Paste	5.00 - 6.77
Smelts, Sauteed	6.67 - 6.90
Soda Crackers	5.65 - 7.32
Soup	
Broccoli Cheese Soup, condensed	5.60
Chicken Broth, rts.	5.80
Corn Soup, condensed	6.80
Cream of Celery Soup, condensed	6.20
Cream of Mushroom, condensed	6.00 - 6.20
Cream style corn, condensed	5.70 - 5.80
Cream of Potato soup, condensed	5.80
Cream of shrimp soup, condensed	5.80
Minestrone condensed	5.40

New England Clam Chowder, condensed	6.00
Oyster Stew, condensed	6.30
Tomato Rice Soup, condensed	5.50
Soy infant formula	6.60 - 7.00
Soy Sauce	4.40 - 5.40
Soybean curd (tofu)	7.20
Soybean milk	7.00
Spaghetti, cooked	5.97 - 6.40
Spinach	5.50 - 6.80
Spinach, chopped	5.38 - 5.52
Spinach, cooked	6.60 - 7.18
Spinach, frozen, cooked	6.30 - 6.52
Spinach, pureed	5.50 - 6.22
Spinach, strained	5.63 - 5.79
Squash, acorn, cooked	5.18 - 6.49
Squash, Kubbard, cooked	6.00 - 6.20
Squash, white, cooked	5.52 - 5.80
Squash, yellow, cooked	5.79 - 6.00
Squid	6.00 - 6.50
Sturgeon	6.20
Strawberries	3.00 -3.90
Strawberries, California	3.32 - 3.50
Strawberries, frozen	3.21 - 3.32
Strawberry Jam	3.00 - 3.40
Straw mushroom	4.90
Sweet Potatoes	5.30 - 5.60
Swiss Chard, cooked	6.17 - 6.78

Tamarind	3.00
Tangerine	3.32 - 4.48
Taro syrup	4.50
Tea	7.20
Three-Bean Salad	5.40
Tofu (soybean Curd)	7.20
Tomatillo (resembling Cherry tomatoes)	3.83
Tomatoes	4.30 - 4.90
Tomatoes, canned	3.50 - 4.70
Tomatoes, Juice	4.10 - 4.60
Tomatoes, Paste	3.50 - 4.70
Tomatoes, Puree	4.30 - 4.47
Tomatoes, Strained	4.32 - 4.58
Tomatoes, Wine ripened	4.42 - 4.65
Tomato Soup, Cream of, canned	4.62
Trout, Sea, sauteed	6.20 - 6.33
Truffle	5.30 - 6.50
Tuna Fish, canned	5.90 - 6.20
Turnips	5.29 - 5.90
Turnip, greens, cooked	5.40 - 6.20
Turnip, white, cooked	5.76 - 5.85
Turnip, yellow, cooked	5.57 - 5.82
Vegetable Juice	3.90 - 4.30
Vegetable soup, canned	5.16
Vegetable soup, chopped	4.98 - 5.02
Vegetable soup, strained	4.99 - 5.0
Vermicelli, cooked	5.80 - 6.50

Vinegar	2.40 - 3.40
Vinegar, cider	3.10
Walnuts, English	5.42
Wax gourd drink	7.20
Water Chestnut	6.00 - 6.20
Watercress	5.88 - 6.18
Watermelon	5.18 - 5.60
Wheat Krispice	4.99 - 5.62
Wheaten	5.85 - 6.08
Wheaties	5.00 - 5.12
Worcestershire sauce	3.63 - 4.00
Yams, cooked	5.50 - 6.81
Yeast	5.65
Yangsberries, frozen	3.00 - 3.70
Zucchini, cooked	5.69 - 6.10
Zwiebach	4.84 - 4.94

BREAKFAST RECIPES

Muesli-Style Oatmeal

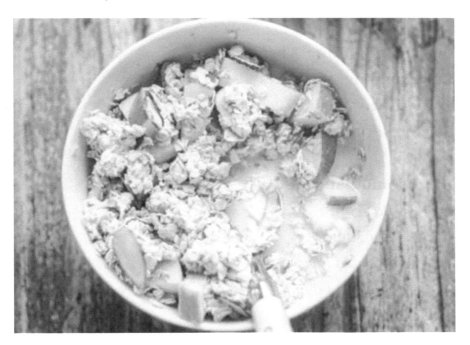

Ingredients:

- 1 cup oatmeal
- 1 cup almond milk
- 2 tablespoons raisins
- 1 apple, peeled, diced
- Pinch of salt
- 2 teaspoon Splenda

How to prepare:

1. Soak oatmeal in milk along with salt, Splenda, and raisins in a glass bowl.

2. Cover and refrigerate the bowl for 2 hours.

3. Stir in apples.

4. Serve.

Preparation time: 5 minutes

Cooking time: 0 minutes

Total time: 5 minutes

Servings: 1

Nutritional Values:

- *Calories 519*
- *Total Fat 31.4 g*
- *Saturated Fat 25.9 g*
- *Cholesterol 0 mg*
- *Sodium 99 mg*
- *Total Carbs 57.8 g*
- *Fiber 8.7 g*
- *Sugar 2.3 g*
- *Protein 6.5 g*

Quinoa Porridge

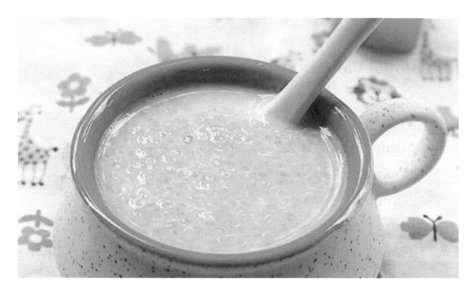

Ingredients:
- ¾ cup quinoa

- 3 cups almond milk

- 3 tablespoons Splenda

- ½ teaspoon vanilla extract

- Salt, to taste

- How to prepare:

- Boil milk in a cooking pot and whisk in quinoa.

- Stir cook the mixture until smooth and creamy.

- Add salt, vanilla, and Splenda.

- Serve.

Preparation time: 5 minutes

Cooking time: 15 minutes

Total time: 20 minutes

Servings: 4

Nutritional Values:

- *Calories 544*
- *Total Fat 24.9 g*
- *Saturated Fat 4.7 g*
- *Cholesterol 194 mg*
- *Sodium 607 mg*
- *Total Carbs 30.7 g*
- *Fiber 1.4 g*
- *Sugar 3.3 g*
- *Protein 6.4g*

Pear Banana Nut Muffins

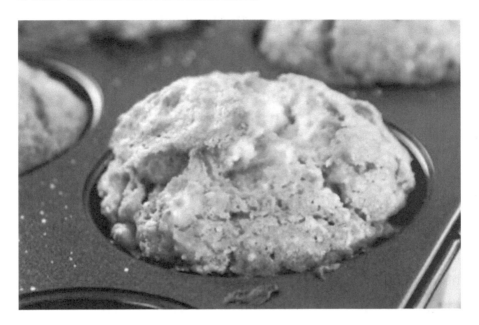

Ingredients:

- 1 medium pear, peeled and diced
- 2 tablespoons pear nectar
- 1 cup coconut flour
- 1 cup rolled oats
- 1 tablespoon ground flaxseed
- 3 tablespoons maple flakes
- 1 teaspoon baking powder
- 1/2 teaspoon baking soda
- 1 teaspoon cinnamon
- 1/4 teaspoon cardamom
- 1/4 teaspoon sea salt
- 2 egg whites

- 1/3 cup vanilla almond milk
- 2 tablespoons almond butter, melted
- 2 teaspoons vanilla
- 1 medium banana, peeled and mashed
- 1 cup chopped walnuts

How to prepare:

1. Set the oven to 375 degrees F. Layer a muffin tray with paper liner and olive oil.
2. Mix pear with pear nectar in a saucepan and boil it.
3. Decrease the heat and cook for 3 minutes. Turn off the heat and allow it to cool.
4. Mix flour with maple flakes, flaxseed, oats, baking soda, baking powder, salt, cinnamon, and cardamom in a bowl.
5. Whisk pear mixture with almond milk, almond butter, vanilla, banana, and egg whites.
6. Stir in flour mixture and mix well.
7. Fold in walnuts and mix well.
8. Divide the mixture into the muffin tray.
9. Bake for 20 minutes.
10. Serve.

Preparation time: 5 minutes
Cooking time: 25 minutes

Total time: 30 minutes

Servings: 8

Nutritional Values:

- *Calories 408*
- *Total Fat 16.5 g*
- *Saturated Fat 5 g*
- *Cholesterol 8 mg*
- *Sodium 285 mg*
- *Total Carbs 56.1 g*
- *Fiber 8.7 g*
- *Sugar 10.1 g*
- *Protein 11 g*

Pumpkin Pancakes

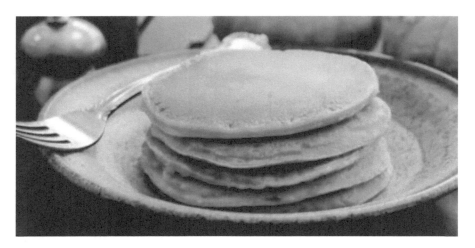

Ingredients:
- 2 cups coconut flour
- 2 tablespoons Splenda
- 1 tablespoon Splenda
- 2 teaspoons baking powder
- 1 teaspoon baking soda
- 1/2 teaspoon salt
- 1 cup pumpkin puree
- 1 teaspoon ground cinnamon
- 1/2 teaspoon ground ginger
- 1/2 teaspoon ground allspice
- 1 egg white
- 1 1/2 cups almond milk
- 2 tablespoons vegetable oil

How to prepare:

1.   Mix flour with sugar, baking powder, soda, salt and Splenda in a large bowl.

2.   Combine pumpkin puree, ginger, cinnamon, allspice, egg whites, milk, and oil in another bowl.

3.   Stir in flour mixture and mix well.

4.   Heat a greased skillet and pour ? cup batter into the pan.

5.   Cook for 3 minutes per side.

6.   Make more pancakes to use the entire batter.

7.   Serve.

Preparation time: 5 minutes
Cooking time: 20 minutes

Total time: 25 minutes

Servings: 6

Nutritional Values:
- *Calories 284*
- *Total Fat 7.9 g*
- *Saturated Fat 0 g*
- *Cholesterol 36 mg*
- *Sodium 704 mg*
- *Total Carbs 46 g*
- *Fiber 3.6 g*
- *Sugar 5.5 g*
- *Protein 7.9 g*

Quick Banana Sorbet

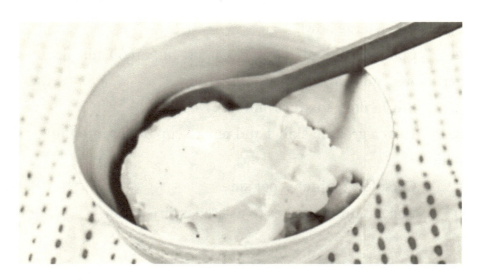

Ingredients:
- 3 bananas, peeled
- 1 tablespoon ginger, peeled and grated fine
- 1/8 teaspoon ground cardamom
- 2 tablespoons honey
- ¼ teaspoon salt
- 3 cups ice

Method:
1.   Blend bananas with cardamom, salt, honey and ginger in a blender.
2.   Stir in ice and blend again until smooth.
3.   Enjoy.

Preparation Time: 5 minutes

Cooking Time: 0 minutes

Total Time: 5 minutes

Servings: 1

Nutritional Values:

- *Calories 462*
- *Total Fat 1.5 g*
- *Saturated Fat 0.5 g*
- *Cholesterol 0 mg*
- *Total Carbs 119.8 g*
- *Dietary Fiber 10 g*
- *Sugar 78 g*
- *Protein 4.5 g*

Oatmeal with Blueberries, Sunflower Seeds

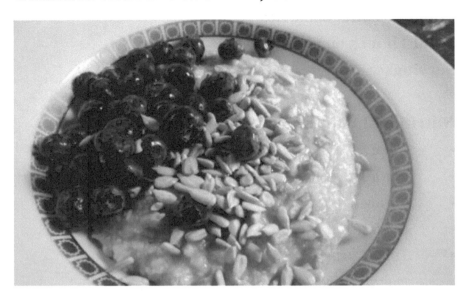

Ingredients:
- 1 serving quick-cooking or old-fashioned rolled oats
- 1/2 cup blueberries
- 1 tablespoon sunflower seeds
- 1 tablespoon agave nectar

How to prepare:
1. Cook oats as per the given instructions on the box.
2. Add blueberries, sunflower seeds, and agave nectar.
3. Serve.

Preparation time: 10 minutes

Cooking time: 25 minutes

Total time: 35 minutes

Servings: 1

Nutritional Values:

- *Calories 134*
- *Total Fat 4.7 g*
- *Saturated Fat 0.6 g*
- *Cholesterol 0 mg*
- *Sodium 1 mg*
- *Total Carbs 54.1 g*
- *Fiber 7 g*
- *Sugar 23.3 g*
- *Protein 6.2 g*

Banana Bread

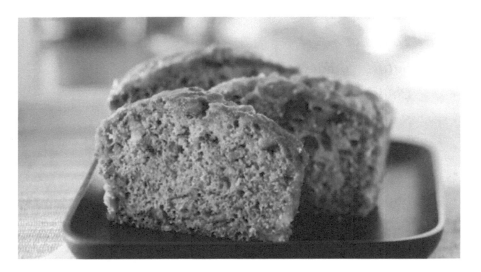

Ingredients:
- 3 bananas, peeled
- 1/3 cup melted almond butter
- 1 teaspoon baking soda
- Pinch of salt
- 3/4 cup Splenda
- 1 egg white, beaten
- 1 teaspoon vanilla extract
- 1 1/2 cups of coconut flour

Method:
1. Adjust your oven to 350 degrees F to preheat.

2. Grease a 4x8 inch bread pan with almond butter.

3. Mash bananas in a glass bowl and whisk in melted almond butter.

4. Mix baking soda with salt in another bowl.

5. Add Splenda, vanilla extract and whisked egg.

6. Stir in flour and mix well until smooth.

7. Transfer the batter into the greased pan.

8. Bake for 50 minutes.

9. Slice and serve.

Preparation Time: 10 minutes

Cooking Time: 50 minutes

Total Time: 60 minutes

Servings: 4

Nutritional Values:

- *Calories 387*
- *Total Fat 6 g*
- *Saturated Fat 9.9 g*
- *Cholesterol 41 mg*
- *Sodium 154 mg*
- *Total Carbs 37.4 g*
- *Fiber 2.9 g*
- *Sugar 15.3 g*
- *Protein 6.6 g*

English Muffins

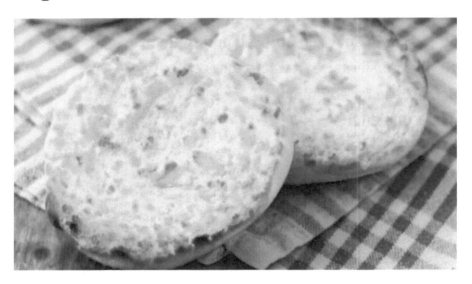

Ingredients:

- 1 3/4 cups almond milk
- 3 tablespoons softened almond butter
- 1 1/2 teaspoons salt, to taste
- 2 tablespoons Splenda
- 1 egg white, lightly beaten
- 4 1/2 cups coconut flour
- 2 teaspoons instant yeast
- Semolina or farina, for sprinkling the griddle or pan

Method:

1. Mix all the muffin ingredients in a mixing bowl except semolina.

2. Blend the ingredients using an electric mixer to form a smooth dough.

3. Let the dough rest for 2 hours.

4.   Grease 2 muffin trays with cooking oil and sprinkle semolina into each cup.

5.   Knead the raised dough and divide it into 16 equal pieces.

6.   Roll each piece into small balls.

7.   Place the balls in the muffin trays and cover them.

8.   Allow them to rest for 20 minutes.

9.   Bake for 15 mins on low heat in the preheated oven until golden.

10.   Serve.

Preparation Time: 10 minutes

Cooking Time: 15 minutes

Total Time: 25 minutes

Servings: 4

Nutritional Values:
- *Calories 212*
- *Total Fat 11.8 g*
- *Saturated Fat 2.2 g*
- *Cholesterol 0 mg*
- *Sodium 321 mg*
- *Total Carbs 14.6 g*
- *Dietary Fiber 4.4 g*
- *Sugar 8 g*
- *Protein 17.3 g*

Steel Cut Oatmeal

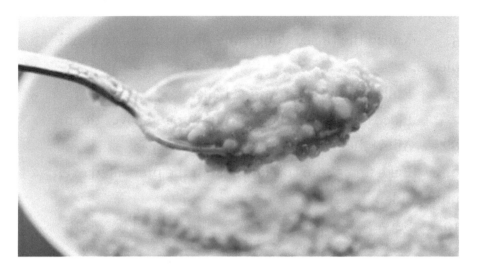

Ingredients:
- 1 tablespoon almond butter
- 1 cup steel cut oats
- 3 cups boiling water
- 1/2 cup almond milk
- 1/2 cup plus 1 tablespoon cashew milk
- 1 tablespoon Splenda
- 1/4 teaspoon cinnamon

Method:

1.   Heat almond butter with oats in a saucepan.

2.   Stir cook for 2 minutes then stirs in boiling water.

3.   Bring the mixture to a low simmer and cook for 25 minutes.

4.   Add half of the almond milk and cashew milk and cook for 10 minutes.

5.   Stir in all the remaining ingredients.

6.   Serve.

Preparation Time: 15 minutes

Cooking Time: 35 minutes

Total Time: 50 minutes

Servings: 1

Nutritional Values:

- *Calories 412*
- *Total Fat 24.8 g*
- *Saturated Fat 12.4 g*
- *Cholesterol 3 mg*
- *Sodium 132 mg*
- *Total Carbs 43.8 g*
- *Dietary Fiber 13.9 g*
- *Sugar 21.5 g*
- *Protein 18.9 g*

Breakfast Porridge

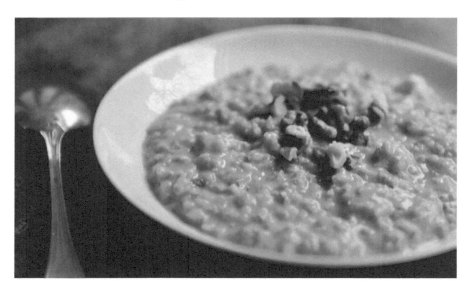

Ingredients:

- 1/2 cup red or wild rice

- 1/2 cup steel-cut oats

- 1/4 cup pearl barley

- 1 cinnamon stick

- 1 to 2 tablespoons Splenda

- 1/4 teaspoon salt

- 1/4 cup dried fruit (cranberries, cherries, raisins)

- Chopped nuts, maple syrup and/or milk, for serving

(optional)

How to prepare:

1.   Soak rice, barley, farina, and oats in 5 cups of water in a rice cooker.

2.   Add cinnamon stick, Splenda, orange peel, salt, and dried fruit.

3.   Cover the cooker and cook for 50 minutes on 'manual' functions.

4.   Serve with nuts on top as desired.

Preparation time: 10 minutes
Cooking time: 50 minutes

Total time: 60 minutes

Servings: 02

Nutritional Values:

- *Calories 331*
- *Total Fat 2.5 g*
- *Saturated Fat 0.5 g*
- *Cholesterol 0 mg*
- *Sodium 595 mg*
- *Total Carbs 69 g*
- *Fiber 12.2 g*
- *Sugar 12.5 g*
- *Protein 8.7g*

APPETIZERS AND SIDES RECIPES

Calm Carrot Salad

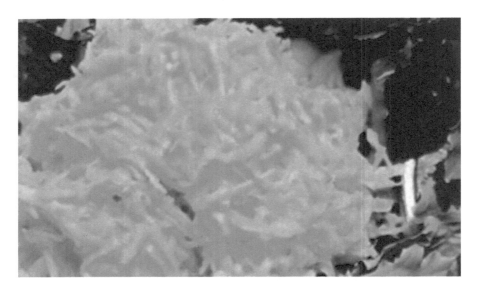

Ingredients:

- 1 lb. carrots (peeled, trimmed, and grated)
- ¼ lb. mesclun greens
- 2 tablespoons raisins
- 1 teaspoon dried oregano
- 2 tablespoons Splenda
- 2 teaspoon olive oil
- ¼ teaspoon salt

How to prepare:

1. Mix oregano, Splenda, salt, raisins, and olive oil in a medium bowl.

2. Toss in carrots and mix well to coat.

3.   Adjust seasoning with salt.

4.   Serve over mesclun greens.

Preparation time: 10 minutes

Cooking time: 0 minutes

Total time: 10 minutes

Servings: 02

Nutritional Values:

- *Calories 144*
- *Total Fat 0.4 g*
- *Saturated Fat 5 g*
- *Cholesterol 51 mg*
- *Sodium 86 mg*
- *Total Carbs 8 g*
- *Fiber 2.3 g*
- *Sugar 2.2 g*
- *Protein 5.6 g*

Chicken Fajita Salad

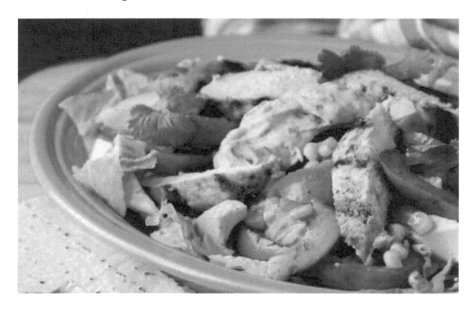

Ingredients:

Marinade/Dressing:
- 3 tablespoons olive oil
- 2 tablespoons cilantro, chopped
- 2 cloves garlic, crushed
- 1 teaspoon Splenda
- 3/4 teaspoon red chili flakes
- 1/2 teaspoon ground Cumin
- 1 teaspoon salt

Salad:
- 4 chicken thigh fillets, skin removed
- 1/2 yellow bell pepper, sliced and deseeded
- 1/2 red bell pepper, deseeded and sliced

- 1/2 an onion, sliced
- 5 cups Romaine, (or cos) lettuce leaves, washed and dried
- 2 avocados, sliced
- Extra cilantro leaves to garnish
- Sour cream, (optional) to serve

How to prepare:

1. To make marinade combine all of its ingredients in a bowl.
2. Season the chicken pieces with this marinade.
3. Marinate the meat for 2 hrs in the refrigerator.
4. Heat a teaspoon of oil in a grill pan. Sear the chicken from sides until golden brown.
5. Transfer the chicken to a plate.
6. Saute onions and pepper in the same pan.
7. Slice the chicken and toss it with pepper, onion, avocado, and leaves in a bowl.
8. Stir in salad dressing.
9. Toss well and serve.

Preparation time: 10 minutes
Cooking time: 5 minutes

Total time: 15 minutes

Servings: 04

Nutritional Values:

- *Calories 184*
- *Total Fat 37 g*
- *Saturated Fat 8 g*
- *Cholesterol 110 mg*
- *Sodium 689 mg*
- *Total Carbs 13 g*
- *Fiber 8 g*
- *Sugar 3 g*
- *Protein 19 g*

Chopped Greek Salad

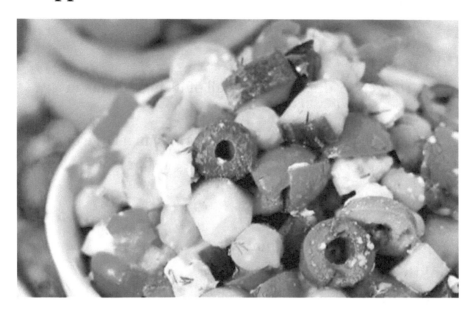

Ingredients:

- 2 cups sliced cucumber
- 1 can chickpeas, drained and rinsed
- 1 cup red bell pepper, diced
- 1/4 cup minced red onion
- 1/2 cup halved kalamata olives
- 1/4 cup of chopped parsley

For the dressing:

- 1/4 cup olive oil
- 1 teaspoon dijon mustard
- 2 tablespoons rice vinegar
- 1/4 teaspoon garlic powder
- 1/4 teaspoon onion powder

- 1/2 teaspoon dried oregano
- Salt and pepper, to taste

How to prepare:

1. To prepare dressing whisk all of its ingredients in a bowl.
2. Toss all the vegetables and chickpeas in a large bowl.
3. Stir in prepared dressing and toss well.
4. Serve.

Preparation time: 10 minutes
Cooking time: 0 minutes
Total time: 10 minutes
Servings: 04

Nutritional Values:

- *Calories 117*
- *Total Fat 13 g*
- *Saturated Fat 3 g*
- *Cholesterol 11 mg*
- *Sodium 332 mg*
- *Total Carbs 4 g*
- *Fiber 1 g*
- *Sugar 2 g*
- *Protein 2 g*

Mediterranean Quinoa Salad

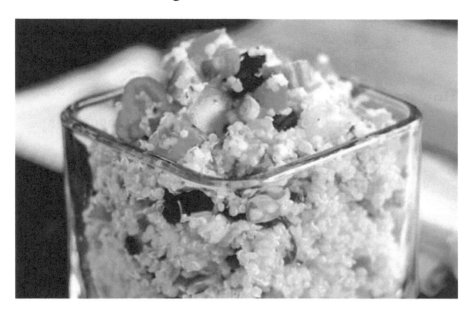

Ingredients:
- 3 cups cooked quinoa
- 1 cup thinly sliced cucumbers
- 1/2 cup diced red bell pepper
- 1/4 cup minced red onion
- 1/4 cup sliced kalamata olives
- 2 tablespoons toasted pine nuts
- 2 tablespoons chopped parsley

For the dressing:
- ¼ cup olive oil
- 1 teaspoon dijon mustard
- 4 tablespoons red wine
- ¼ teaspoon garlic powder

- ¼ teaspoon onion powder
- ½ teaspoon dried oregano
- Salt and pepper, to taste

How to prepare:

1. To prepare dressing, whisk all of its ingredients in a bowl.
2. Toss all the vegetables and quinoa in a large bowl.
3. Stir in prepared dressing and toss well.
4. Serve.

Preparation time: 10 minutes
Cooking time: 0 minutes
Total time: 10 minutes
Servings: 04

Nutritional Values:

- *Calories 307*
- *Total Fat 25 g*
- *Saturated Fat 5 g*
- *Cholesterol 16 mg*
- *Sodium 372 mg*
- *Total Carbs 16 g*
- *Fiber 5 g*
- *Sugar 4 g*
- *Protein 10 g*

Kale and Quinoa Salad

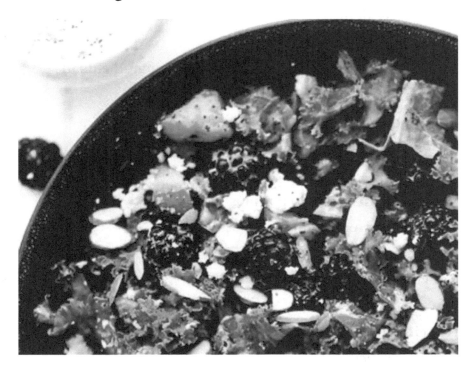

Ingredients:

- 1/2 cup cooked red quinoa
- 6-8 leaves kale washed and trimmed
- 1 teaspoon coarse sea salt
- 3/4 cup fresh strawberries, sliced
- 3/4 cup fresh blackberries
- 3/4 cup fresh raspberries
- 1/2 cup red grapes, halved
- 1/3 cup dried blueberries
- 1/4 cup pistachios, coarsely chopped
- 1 tablespoon olive oil
- Black pepper to taste

How to prepare:

1.   Toss all the vegetables, fruits and quinoa in a large bowl.

2.   For dressing, mix all the remaining ingredients in another bowl.

3.   Add this mixture to the salad.

4.   Mix well and serve.

Preparation time: 10 minutes

Cooking time: 0 minutes

Total time: 10 minutes

Servings: 04

Nutritional Values:

- *Calories 334*
- *Total Fat 1.3 g*
- *Saturated Fat 5 g*
- *Cholesterol 31 mg*
- *Sodium 86 mg*
- *Total Carbs 8 g*
- *Fiber 2.3 g*
- *Sugar 2.2 g*
- *Protein 4.6 g*

Crispy Chicken Tenders

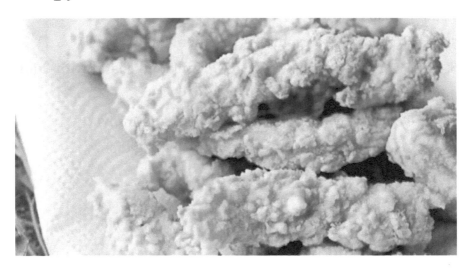

Ingredients:
- 1 pound chicken tenders
- 1 cup almond milk
- 1 tablespoon canola oil
- 3/4 cup coconut flour
- 1/2 teaspoon fresh cracked black pepper
- 1/2 teaspoon salt
- 1 cup panko breadcrumbs
- Canola cooking spray

How to prepare:
1. Soak chicken in the almond milk in a glass bowl.

2. Cover the bowl and refrigerate for 30 minutes.

3. Meanwhile, set the oven to 400 degrees F. Grease a baking dish with canola oil.

4.   Combine flour with cayenne pepper, salt, and pepper in a shallow glass bowl.

5.   Spread panko crumbs in another shallow bowl.

6.   Remove the chicken from the milk and coat it with flour mixture.

7.   Place the coated chicken in the breadcrumbs.

8.   Arrange the coated pieces in the baking dish.

9.   Bake for 25 minutes.

10. Serve warm.

Preparation time: 10 minutes
Cooking time: 35 minutes
Total time: 45 minutes
Servings: 04

Nutritional Values:
- *Calories 124*
- *Total Fat 3.5 g*
- *Saturated Fat 7 g*
- *Cholesterol 51 mg*
- *Sodium 86 mg*
- *Total Carbs 7.5 g*
- *Fiber 2.3 g*
- *Sugar 2.2 g*
- *Protein 14.5 g*

Stuffed Fat Free Potatoes

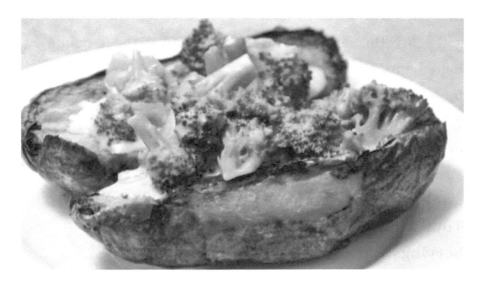

Ingredients:

- 1 pound of turkey breast
- 4 baking potatoes, baked
- 1 pkg. frozen chopped spinach, thawed & drained
- 1/2 to 3/4 cup nonfat cottage cheese
- 2 to 3 tablespoons unflavored yogurt
- 8 ounces of frozen broccoli
- Salt and pepper, to taste

How to prepare:

1. Preheat the oven to 350 degrees F.

2. Dice the turkey in cubes. Saute the cubes in a pan until al dente.

3. Bake all the potatoes for 10 to 15 minutes in the preheated oven.

4.   Slice the potatoes in half then scoop out the flesh from the center.

5.   Mix this flesh with turkey cubes and all the remaining ingredients.

6.   Stuff the potatoes with this mixture.

7.   Serve.

Preparation time: 10 minutes

Cooking time: 20 minutes

Total time: 30 minutes

Servings: 04

Nutritional Values:

- Calories 221
- Total Fat 12.4 g
- Saturated Fat 5 g
- Cholesterol 61 mg
- Sodium 216 mg
- Total Carbs 28 g
- Fiber 2.3 g
- Sugar 1.2 g
- Protein 7.6 g

Carrot Fries

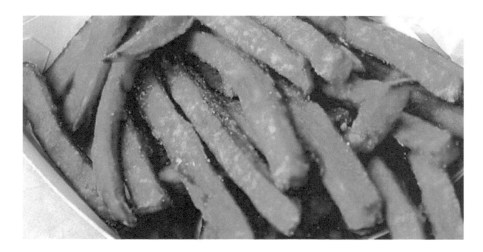

Ingredients:
- 1-1/2 pounds carrots, scrubbed and cut into sticks
- 1 tablespoon olive oil
- 1 tablespoon fresh rosemary, finely chopped
- Salt and pepper, to taste
- How to prepare:
- Set the oven to 425 degrees F to preheat.
- Toss carrots with the all ingredients in a bowl to coat.
- Spread the carrots in a baking pan.
- Bake for 30 minutes.
- Serve warm.

Preparation time: 10 minutes

Cooking time: 30 minutes

Total time: 40 minutes

Servings: 04

Nutritional Values:

- *Calories 153*
- *Total Fat 2.4 g*
- *Saturated Fat 3 g*
- *Cholesterol 21 mg*
- *Sodium 216 mg*
- *Total Carbs 8 g*
- *Fiber 2.3 g*
- *Sugar 1.2 g*
- *Protein 3.2 g*

Millet Cauliflower Mash

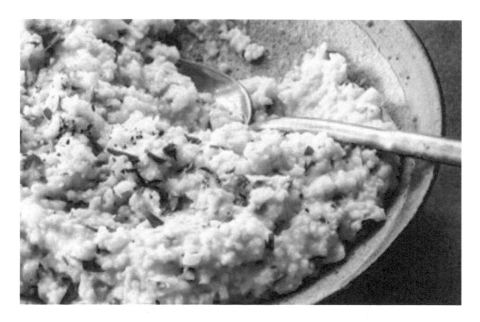

Ingredients:

- 1 cup millet
- 3 cups water
- 1 cup cauliflower florets
- 1/4 teaspoon salt
- 1 teaspoon tamari
- Sprig of parsley, for garnish

How to prepare:

1. Roast the millet in a nonstick pan for 5 minutes.

2. Boil water in a large pan on high heat then add cauliflower, salt, and millet.

3. Cover the dish with the lid then cook for 25 minutes on low heat.

4. Stir in tamari and cook for 5 minutes.

5. Lightly mash the cauliflower mixture.

6. Garnish with parsley and serve.

Preparation time: 10 minutes

Cooking time: 30 minutes

Total time: 40 minutes

Servings: 04

Nutritional Values:

- *Calories 454*
- *Total Fat 4 g*
- *Saturated Fat 5 g*
- *Cholesterol 0 mg*
- *Sodium 233 mg*
- *Total Carbs 30 g*
- *Fiber 6 g*
- *Sugar 2.2 g*
- *Protein 4 g*

Sauteed Swiss Chard

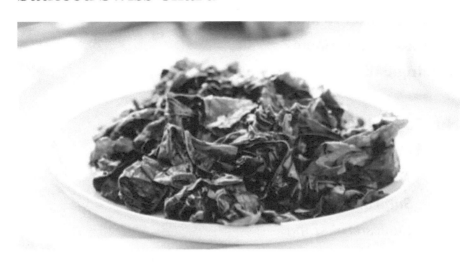

Ingredients:
- 2 tablespoons pine nuts
- 1 tablespoon olive oil
- 1 bunch Swiss chard, stems trimmed, leaves chopped
- 2 tablespoons golden raisins
- 1/8 teaspoon thyme
- Salt and pepper, to taste

How to prepare:
1. Toast the pine nuts for 4 minutes in the nonstick skillet.
2. Transfer the pine nuts to a plate and set them aside.
3. Heat olive oil in the same pan.
4. Stir in thyme, swiss chard, and raisins.
5. Saute for 5 minutes and adjust seasoning with salt and pepper.
6. Serve with pine nuts on top.

Preparation time: 10 minutes

Cooking time: 10 minutes

Total time: 20 minutes

Servings: 02

Nutritional Values:

- *Calories 167*
- *Total Fat 2.4 g*
- *Saturated Fat 5 g*
- *Cholesterol 51 mg*
- *Sodium 86 mg*
- *Total Carbs 4.2 g*
- *Fiber 2.3 g*
- *Sugar 2.2 g*
- *Protein 5.6 g*

VEGETARIAN AND VEGAN RECIPES

Seitan & Black Bean Stir-Fry

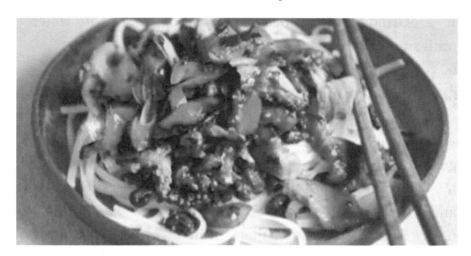

Ingredients:
- 3/4 lb. can black beans, drained and rinsed
- 1 tablespoon Splenda
- 3 garlic cloves
- 2 tablespoons soy sauce
- 1 teaspoon Chinese five-spice powder
- 2 tablespoons rice vinegar
- 1 tablespoon smooth peanut almond butter
- 1 red chili, finely chopped

For the stir-fry
- 2/3 lb. jar marinated seitan pieces
- 1 tablespoon xanthan gum
- 2-3 tablespoon vegetable oil
- 1 red pepper, sliced
- 2/3 lb. bok choy, chopped

- 2 spring onions, sliced
- Cooked rice noodles or rice, to serve

How to prepare:
1.   Grind half of the beans in a food processor with water until smooth.
2.   Drain seitan and pat it dry.
3.   Toss the seitan with xanthan gum in a bowl and set it aside.
4.   Heat oil in a skillet and saute seitan for 5 minutes until golden brown.
5.   Stir in shallots, peppers, remaining beans, spring onion, and bok choy.
6.   Saute for 4 minutes then stir in the blended sauce.
7.   Boil for 1 minute then serves with rice.

Preparation time: 5 minutes
Cooking time: 10 minutes
Total time: 15 minutes
Servings: 04

Nutritional Values:
- *Calories 383*
- *Total Fat 5.3 g*
- *Saturated Fat 3.9 g*
- *Cholesterol 135 mg*
- *Sodium 487 mg*
- *Total Carbs 76.8 g*
- *Fibre 0.1g*
- *Sugar 0 g*
- *Protein 17.7 g*

Stir-fried Garlic Green Beans

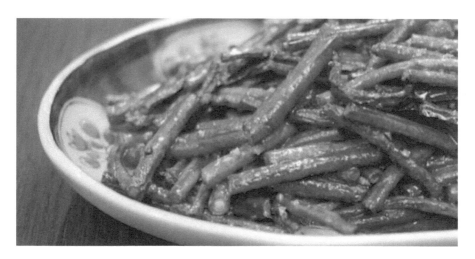

Ingredients:
- 2 tablespoons sunflower oil
- ½ lb. pack trimmed green beans
- 3 garlic cloves, finely sliced
- 1 teaspoon oyster sauce or soy sauce

How to prepare:
1. Preheat oil in a skillet and add green beans.
2. Saute for 5 minutes then stir in garlic.
3. Add oyster sauce and saute for 2 minutes.
4. Serve.

Preparation time: 5 minutes
Cooking time: 10 minutes

Total time: 15 minutes

Servings: 2

Nutritional Values:

- *Calories 198*
- *Total Fat 3.8 g*
- *Saturated Fat 5.1 g*
- *Cholesterol 20 mg*
- *Sodium 272 mg*
- *Total Carbs 3.6 g*
- *Fiber 1 g*
- *Sugar 1.3 g*
- *Protein 1.8 g*

Tenderstem Broccoli

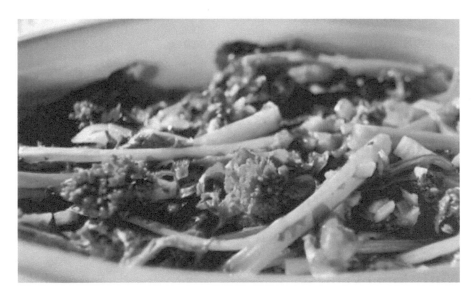

Ingredients:
- ¼ cup whole blanched peanuts
- 2 tablespoons olive oil
- 1 banana shallot, thinly sliced
- 2/3 lb. broccoli, trimmed and cut into florets
- ¼ red pepper, cut into thin strips
- ½ yellow pepper, cut into thin strips
- 2 tablespoons oyster sauce

How to prepare:
1. Set the oven to 284 degrees F to preheat.
2. Spread the nuts in a baking sheet in a single layer and roast for 15 minutes.
3. Heat oil in an iron wok and stir in shallots.

4. Saute for 10 minutes until golden brown.

5. Add peppers and broccoli. Stir cook for 3 minutes.

6. Stir in water, salt, and oyster sauce.

7. Cook for 5 minutes.

8. Garnish with peanuts and serve warm.

Preparation time: 10 minutes

Cooking time: 20 minutes

Total time: 30 minutes

Servings: 2

Nutritional Values:

- *Calories 372*
- *Total Fat 11.8 g*
- *Saturated Fat 4.4 g*
- *Cholesterol 62 mg*
- *Sodium 871 mg*
- *Total Carbs 11.8 g*
- *Fiber 0.6 g*
- *Sugar 7.3 g*
- *Protein 4 g*

Gingered Tofu, Aubergine & Pea Noodles

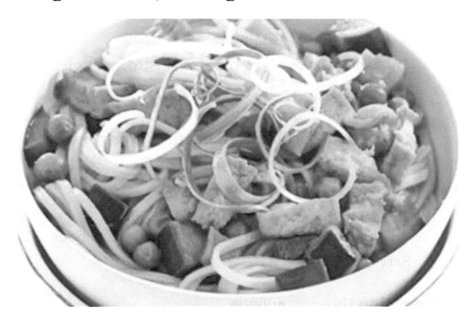

Ingredients:

- 3 tablespoon toasted sesame oil
- 2 aubergines, cut into small chunks
- 4 nests medium egg noodles
- 1 garlic clove
- 1 thumb-sized piece ginger, grated
- 2 teaspoon Chinese five-spice powder
- 3 tablespoon soy sauce
- 3 tablespoons sweet chili sauce
- 1 (1/4 lb.) pack marinated tofu pieces
- ½ cup frozen peas, defrosted
- 3 spring onions, shredded

How to prepare:

1. Heat a greased skillet and add aubergine to saute for 10 minutes while adding seasonings.

2. Cook the noodles as per the given instructions on the box until al dente.

3. Transfer the aubergine to a plate.

4. Pour oil into the same pan and stir in ginger and garlic.

5. Saute for 30 seconds then add five spice.

6. Stir in chili sauce and soy sauce. Cook for 30 seconds.

7. Toss in tofu, aubergines, and peas. Mix well.

8. Add boiled noodles and garnish with spring onions.

9. Serve.

Preparation time: 10 minutes
Cooking time: 30 minutes

Total time: 40 minutes

Servings: 4

Nutritional Values:

- *Calories 341*
- *Total Fat 4 g*
- *Saturated Fat 0.5 g*
- *Cholesterol 69 mg*
- *Sodium 547 mg*
- *Total Carbs 16.4 g*
- *Fiber 1.2 g*
- *Sugar 1 g*
- *Protein 0.3 g*

Sesame Spinach

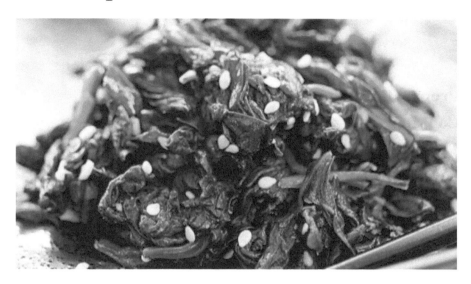

Ingredients:

- 1 tablespoon toasted sesame oil
- ½ tablespoon soy sauce
- ½ teaspoon toasted sesame seeds, crushed
- ½ teaspoon Splenda
- 1 garlic clove, grated
- 1 cup spinach, stem ends trimmed

How to prepare:

1. Boil water in a pot then add spinach for 1 minute until it is wilted.

2. Strain the spinach and set it aside.

3. Mix sesame oil, sesame seeds, soy sauce, Splenda, pepper, and garlic in a bowl.

4.   Toss the parboiled spinach with prepared dressing in a large glass bowl.

5.   Serve.

Preparation time: 10 minutes
Cooking time: 5 minutes
Total time: 15 minutes
Servings: 01

Nutritional Values:
- *Calories 311*
- *Total Fat 0.5 g*
- *Saturated Fat 2.4 g*
- *Cholesterol 69 mg*
- *Sodium 58 mg*
- *Total Carbs 1.4 g*
- *Fiber 0.7 g*
- *Sugar 0.3 g*
- *Protein 1.4 g*

Potato Medley Soup

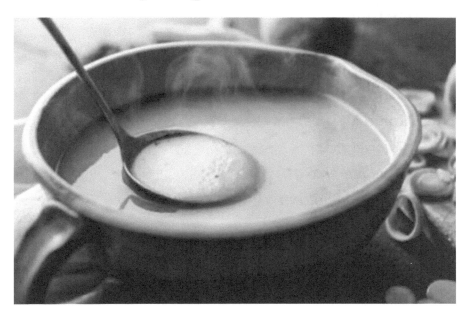

Ingredients:
- ½ lb. chopped raw vegetables, such as onions, celery, and carrots
- 2/3 lb. potato
- 1 tablespoon oil
- 3 cups stock
- Fresh herbs, to serve

How to prepare:
1. Saute vegetables with potatoes in a greased cooking pot until soft.
2. Stir in stock and bring it to a simmer.
3. Cook for 15 minutes then blend until smooth.
4. Serve warm with fresh herbs on top.

Preparation time: 10 minutes

Cooking time: 15 minutes

Total time: 25 minutes

Servings:

Nutritional Values:

- *Calories 304*
- *Total Fat 30.6 g*
- *Saturated Fat 13.1 g*
- *Cholesterol 131 mg*
- *Sodium 834 mg*
- *Total Carbs 21.4g*
- *Fiber 0.2 g*
- *Sugar 0.3 g*
- *Protein 4.6 g*

Vegetable Soup

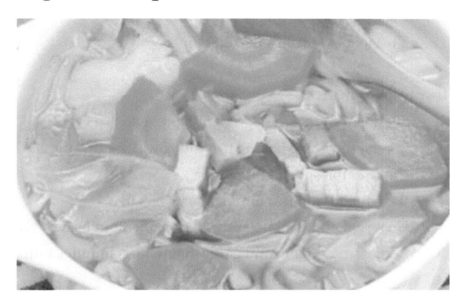

Ingredients:

- ½ lb. sourdough bread, cut into croutons
- 1 tablespoon caraway seeds
- 3 tablespoons olive oil
- 1 garlic clove, chopped
- 1 carrot, chopped
- 1 potato, chopped
- 3 cups vegetable stock
- Pinch of golden caster sugar
- 2 bay leaves
- 1 rosemary sprig
- 2 thyme sprigs
- 1 celery stick, chopped
- ½ lb. cauliflower, cut into florets

- ¼ lb. white cabbage, shredded
- 1 teaspoon Worcestershire sauce
- 2 teaspoons mushroom ketchup

How to prepare:

1. Set the oven to 320 degrees F to preheat.

2. Spread the bread baking tray along with caraway seeds, sea salt, and 1 tablespoon oil.

3. Bake for 10 minutes until golden.

4. Heat remaining oil in large pot over medium heat.

5. Add carrot, potato, and garlic. Saute for 5 minutes until soft.

6. Stir in celery, seasoning, sugar, stock, bay leaves, thyme, and rosemary.

7. Boil the mixture then reduce the heat to a simmer.

8. Cook for 10 minutes then add cabbage and cauliflower.

9. Cook for another 15 minutes until al dente.

10. Stir in mushroom ketchup and Worcestershire sauce.

11. Discard bay leaves, thyme, and rosemary and serve warm.

Preparation time: 10 minutes
Cooking time: 40 minutes
Total time: 50 minutes
Servings: 04

Nutritional Values:

- Calories 418
- Total Fat 3.8 g
- Saturated Fat 0.7 g
- Cholesterol 2 mg
- Sodium 620 mg
- Total Carbs 13.3 g
- Fiber 2.4 g
- Sugar 1.2 g
- Protein 5.4 g

Spiced Parsnip Soup

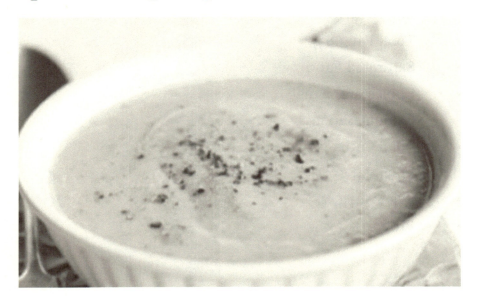

Ingredients:

- 2 garlic cloves, sliced
- 1 small piece ginger, peeled and sliced
- 1 onion, sliced
- 6 parsnips, peeled and chopped
- 1 teaspoon cumin seed
- 1 teaspoon coriander seed
- 2 cardamom pods
- 2 tablespoons almond butter
- 1 tablespoon garam masala
- 5 cups vegetable stock
- ¼ cup coconut cream

To serve

- 1 teaspoon olive oil
- 1 teaspoon toasted cumin seeds

- 1 red chili, deseeded and sliced
- Coriander leaves

How to prepare:

1. Melt almond butter in a cooking pot and add onion to saute until soft.

2. Stir in ginger and garlic. Saute for 1 minute.

3. Add spices and parsnips. Stir cook for 3 minutes.

4. Stir in stock and cook for 30 minutes.

5. Add cream and bring the soup to a boil then turn off the heat.

6. Puree the soup using a handheld blender.

7. Serve warm with desired toppings.

Preparation time: 10 minutes
Cooking time: 30 minutes

Total time: 40 minutes

Servings: 04

Nutritional Values:
- *Calories 438*
- *Total Fat 4.8 g*
- *Saturated Fat 1.7 g*
- *Cholesterol 12 mg*
- *Sodium 520 mg*
- *Total Carbs 58.3 g*
- *Fiber 2.3 g*
- *Sugar 1.2 g*
- *Protein 2.2g*

Almond Butternut Squash & Sage Risotto

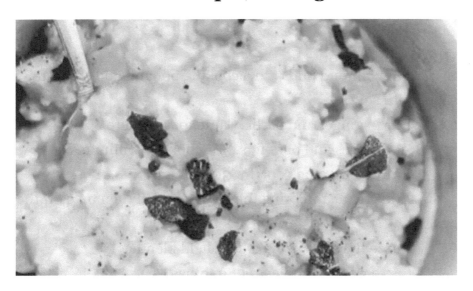

Ingredients:

- 2 lbs. butternut squash, peeled and cut into pieces
- 3 tablespoon olive oil
- 1 bunch sage, half roughly chopped, half whole
- 5 ½ cups vegetable stock
- ¼ cup almond butter
- 1 onion, finely chopped
- 2/3 lb. brown rice
- 1 small glass white wine
- Vegetarian alternative, finely grated

How to prepare:

1. Adjust the oven to 350 degrees F.

2. Toss squash with 1 tablespoon oil and sage in a baking sheet.

3.   Roast for 30 minutes until soft and brown.

4.   Heat half of the almond butter in a pan and add onions to saute for 10 minutes.

5.   Add rice and saute for 3 to 5 minutes.

6.   Stir in wine and let it simmer.

7.   Pour in boiled stock and cook for 25 minutes until rice is al dente.

8.   Puree the risotto using a handheld blender.

9.   Stir in roasted almond butter squash mixture.

10.   Serve warm.

Preparation time: 10 minutes

Cooking time: 60 minutes

Total time: 1 hour 10 minutes

Servings: 06

Nutritional Values:
- *Calories 246*
- *Total Fat 14.8 g*
- *Saturated Fat 0.7 g*
- *Cholesterol 22 mg*
- *Sodium 220 mg*
- *Total Carbs 40.3 g*
- *Fiber 2.4 g*
- *Sugar 1.2 g*
- *Protein 12.4g*

Mushroom & Spinach Risotto

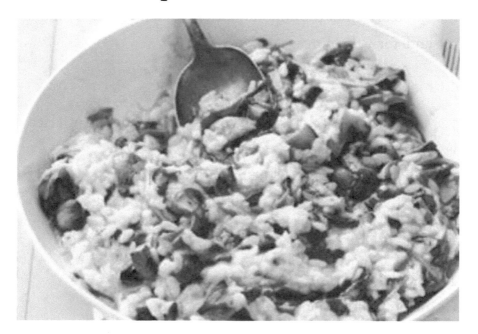

Ingredients:

- 1 tablespoon olive oil
- 1 tablespoon almond butter
- 1 onion, chopped
- ¼ cup chestnut mushrooms, sliced
- 1 garlic clove, crushed
- 2/3 cup brown rice
- ½ cup dry white wine
- 2 cups hot vegetable stock
- 2 tablespoon chopped fresh parsley
- Vegetarian alternative, freshly grated
- 1 cup fresh young leaf spinach, washed if necessary
- Warm ciabatta and green salad, to serve

How to prepare:

1.   Heat almond butter and oil in a large cooking pot and onion to saute for 5 minutes.

2.   Add garlic and mushrooms and stir cook for 3 minutes.

3.   Stir in rice and wine then cook for 3 minutes.

4.   Pour in stock and cook until it is entirely absorbed.

5.   Add parsley, seasoning, and spinach.

6.   Cover the dish with the lid then cook for 5 minutes.

7.   Serve warm.

Preparation time: 10 minutes

Cooking time: 20 minutes

Total time: 30 minutes

Servings: 04

Nutritional Values:

- *Calories 338*
- *Total Fat 3.8 g*
- *Saturated Fat 0.7 g*
- *Cholesterol 22 mg*
- *Sodium 620 mg*
- *Total Carbs 58.3 g*
- *Fiber 2.4 g*
- *Sugar 1.2 g*
- *Protein 5.4g*

SEAFOOD AND POULTRY RECIPES

Seared Salmon with Sauteed Summer Vegetables

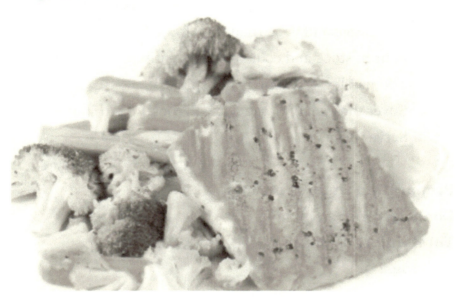

Ingredients:

- 1 red bell pepper, chopped
- 1 tablespoon olive oil
- 3 cups broccoli florets
- 1 carrot, peeled and sliced
- 1 yellow bell pepper, diced
- 1 cucumber, peeled and cut into spears
- 5 radishes, quartered
- 4 basil leaves, chopped
- 1/4 teaspoon salt
- 1 teaspoon coconut oil
- Four 5-ounce salmon fillets

How to prepare:

1.   Boil water in a cooking pot and steam the broccoli florets in the pot for 6 minutes.

2.   Heat oil in a nonstick pan then add carrots.

3.   Saute for 3 minutes then stir in broccoli, radishes, cucumber, and peppers.

4.   Stir cook for 3 minutes then seasons with salt and basil.

5.   Transfer the veggies mixture to a bowl.

6.   Heat coconut oil in the same pan over medium heat.

7.   Sear the salmon for 4 minutes per side. Season it with salt and pepper.

8.   Serve the salmon with vegetables.

Preparation time: 10 minutes
Cooking time: 20 minutes

Total time: 30 minutes

Servings: 04

Nutritional Values:

- *Calories 272*
- *Total Fat 11 g*
- *Saturated Fat 3 g*
- *Cholesterol 66 mg*
- *Sodium 288 mg*
- *Total Carbs 10 g*
- *Fibre 4g*
- *Sugar 0 g*
- *Protein 33 g*

Coconut Panko Shrimp

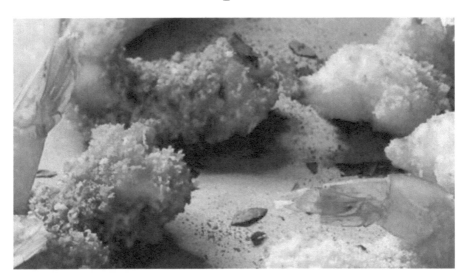

Ingredients:

- 1/2 cup panko flakes
- 1 4-ounce bag coconut flakes
- 2 lb. large shrimp, deveined
- 4 eggs, white
- 1 cup coconut oil

How to prepare:

1. Mix panko with coconut flakes in a shallow bowl.

2. Beat egg whites in another bowl.

3. Dip the shrimps the egg whites then coat with crumbs mixture.

4. Arrange the shrimps in a greased baking sheet.

5. Bake for about 10 to 15 minutes until al dente.

6. Serve warm.

Preparation time: 10 minutes

Cooking time: 15 minutes

Total time: 25 minutes

Servings: 4

Nutritional Values:

- *Calories 557*
- *Total Fat 29 g*
- *Saturated Fat 22 g*
- *Cholesterol 550 mg*
- *Sodium 1800 mg*
- *Total Carbs 25 g*
- *Fiber 3 g*
- *Sugar 0.3 g*
- *Protein 47 g*

Coconut Cod Fish

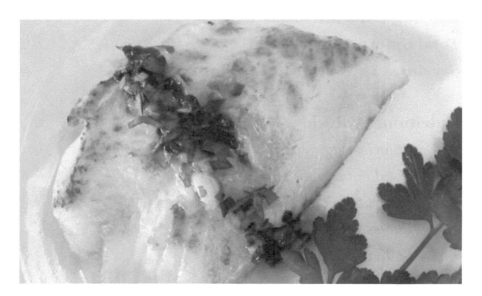

Ingredients:
- 2 cod fish fillets
- 1⁄2 cup coconut milk
- Salt and pepper, to taste
- 2 sheets kitchen aluminum foil
- 1 tablespoon dried herbs

How to prepare:
- Set the oven to 350 degrees F.
- Place the fish fillets on foil sheets.
- Drizzle herbs and seasonings over the fish.
- Partially cover the fish with foil sheet to make a nest.
- Divide milk into each foil nest.

- Seal the nest and bake for 20 minutes.
- Serve warm.

Preparation time: 5 minutes

Cooking time: 20 minutes

Total time: 25 minutes

Servings: 2

Nutritional Values:
- *Calories 301*
- *Total Fat 12.2 g*
- *Saturated Fat 2.4 g*
- *Cholesterol 110 mg*
- *Sodium 276 mg*
- *Total Carbs 5 g*
- *Fiber 0.9 g*
- *Sugar 1.4 g*
- *Protein 28.8 g*

Fish Fillets in Parchment

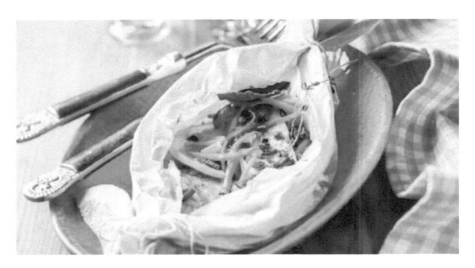

Ingredients:

- 4-ounce halibut fillets
- 1/4 cup chopped fresh broccoli
- 1 tablespoon whole capers
- 1 small red potato chopped
- 1/4 cup julienne cut carrot
- A few herbs such as parsley, cilantro or basil
- 1 tablespoon olive oil
- Black pepper

How to prepare:

1. Set the oven to 450 degrees F to preheat.

2. Cut a 14 inch square of parchment paper and fold it into a triangle.

3. Place the fillets at the center of the fold.

4.	Top the fish with remaining ingredients, herbs, and olive oil.

5.	Wrap the fish with parchment paper and place them in a baking sheet.

6.	Bake for 15 minutes.

7.	Serve warm.

Preparation time: 5 minutes

Cooking time: 15 minutes

Total time: 20 minutes

Servings: 4

Nutritional Values:

- *Calories 310*
- *Total Fat 2.4 g*
- *Saturated Fat 0.1 g*
- *Cholesterol 320 mg*
- *Sodium 350 mg*
- *Total Carbs 12.2 g*
- *Fiber 0.7 g*
- *Sugar 0.7 g*
- *Protein 44.3 g*

Baked Herb Tilapia

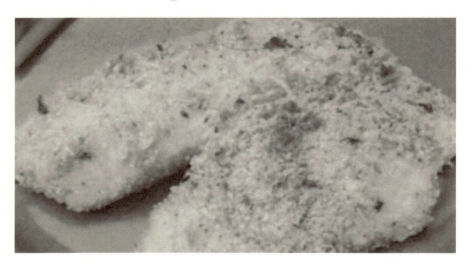

Ingredients:
- Olive oil spray
- 2 tilapia fillets
- Dried basil
- Dried oregano
- Dried thyme
- Sea salt

How to prepare:

1.   Set the oven to 350 degrees F.

2.   Layer a baking sheet with foil and olive oil.

3.   Arrange the fish in the baking sheet and top it with herbs, salt, and olive oil.

4.   Bake for 15 minutes.

5.   Serve.

Preparation time: 5 minutes

Cooking time: 1 hour 30 minutes

Total time: 1 hour 35 minutes

Servings: 06

Nutritional Values:

- *Calories 372*
- *Total Fat 1.1 g*
- *Saturated Fat 3.8 g*
- *Cholesterol 10 mg*
- *Sodium 749 mg*
- *Total Carbs 4.9 g*
- *Fiber 0.2 g*
- *Sugar 0.2 g*
- *Protein 33.5 g*

Asian Peanut Chicken with Noodles

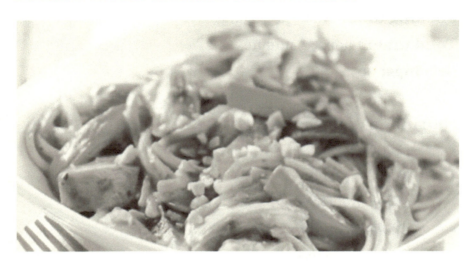

Ingredients:
- 3 quarts water
- 3 tablespoon smooth peanut almond butter
- 1/4 cup fresh cilantro leaves
- 2 teaspoon low-sodium soy sauce
- 4 tablespoon low sodium chicken or vegetable broth
- 1/8 teaspoon red pepper flakes
- 6 ounces boneless skinless chicken breast, sliced into strips
- 1/2 cup frozen edamame soybeans
- 4 ounces whole wheat or gluten-free spaghetti
- 1 small carrot, shredded
- 1 onion, sliced
- 2 tablespoons dry roasted unsalted peanuts

How to prepare:
1. Blend peanut almond butter, stock, red pepper, soy sauce, and cilantro in a blender.

2. Set the oven to 200 degrees F to preheat.

3. Boil 3 quarts water in a pan then add chicken to cook for 5 minutes.

4. Transfer the chicken to a baking pan using a slotted spoon.

5. Boil the remaining cooking water and add pasta into it.

6. Cook for 10 minutes until al dente and add edamame to cook for 1 minute.

7. Reserve half cup of the cooking liquid.

8. Drain the edamame and pasta.

9. Add the pasta, edamame to a pan along with chicken, carrots, and peanut sauce.

10. Stir cook for 1 minute and add reserved liquid to achieve the desired consistency.

11. Serve warm.

Preparation time: 5 minutes
Cooking time: 15 minutes
Total time: 20 minutes
Servings: 2

Nutritional Values:
- *Calories 581*
- *Total Fat 23 g*
- *Saturated Fat 4 g*
- *Cholesterol 49 mg*
- *Sodium 257 mg*
- *Total Carbs 3.6g*
- *Fiber 10 g*
- *Sugar 0.5 g*
- *Protein 58 g*

Cashew Chicken

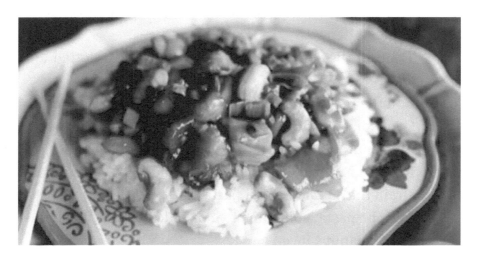

Ingredients:

- 1 lb chicken breast, cut into strips
- 1/2 cup vegetable broth
- 1 cup frozen shelled edamame soybeans
- 2 teaspoon sesame oil
- 2 cups water
- 1 cup brown rice uncooked
- 1 white onion diced
- 1 tablespoon ginger, minced
- 2 tablespoon low-sodium soy sauce
- 1 garlic clove,minced
- 1/2 cup raw cashews
- 1 tablespoon maple syrup

How to prepare:

1. Heat water in a pan then add rice. Cook for 25 minutes on low flame.

2. Put off the heat and strain the rice.

3. Heat a tsp sesame oil in a skillet and add onion.

4. Saute for 5 to 10 minutes until soft then set it aside.

5. Heat more sesame oil in the same pan and add garlic.

6. Cook until light brown.

7. Stir in cashews, ginger, and chicken. Stir cook for 5 minutes.

8. Pour in maple syrup, soy sauce, and broth.

9. Stir in onions and cook for 5 minutes.

10. Add edamame and cook for 8 minutes.

11. Serve with boiled rice.

Preparation time: 5 minutes
Cooking time: 55 minutes

Total time: 60 minutes

Servings: 4

Nutritional Values:
- *Calories 529*
- *Total Fat 17 g*
- *Saturated Fat 3 g*
- *Cholesterol 65 mg*
- *Sodium 391 mg*
- *Total Carbs 55 g*
- *Fiber 6 g*
- *Sugar 8 g*
- *Protein 41g*

Chicken Fajitas with Roasted Red Peppers

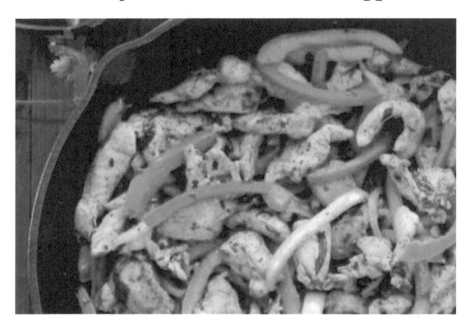

Ingredients:

- 1 white onion, peeled and sliced thin
- 1 quarts water
- 1 red bell pepper
- spray olive oil
- 2/3 lb. chicken breast, slice into thin strips
- 1/4 teaspoon salt
- 1/4 teaspoon ground cumin
- 1/4 cup water
- 4 chickpea flour tortillas
- 1 tablespoon fresh cilantro leaves (per serving)

How to prepare:

1. Adjust the oven to 350 degrees F.

2.   Spread the red pepper in a baking sheet and bake for 40 minutes.

3.   Keep tossing the pepper after every 10 minutes.

4.   Let the peppers cool down then peel off the skin and slice it.

5.   Heat a greased skillet and add onions to saute until brown.

6.   Stir in sliced pepper, chicken, cumin, and salt.

7.   Saute for 5 to 10 minutes until chicken is lightly browned.

8.   Pour in water and cook on high heat until only 1 tablespoon liquid is left.

9.   Serve the fajita with a warm tortilla.

Preparation time: 10 minutes
Cooking time: 60 minutes
Total time: 70 minutes
Servings: 4

Nutritional Values:
- *Calories 284*
- *Total Fat 25 g*
- *Saturated Fat 1 g*
- *Cholesterol 49 mg*
- *Sodium 460 mg*
- *Total Carbs 35 g*
- *Fiber 2 g*
- *Sugar 6 g*
- *Protein 26g*

Chicken Satay

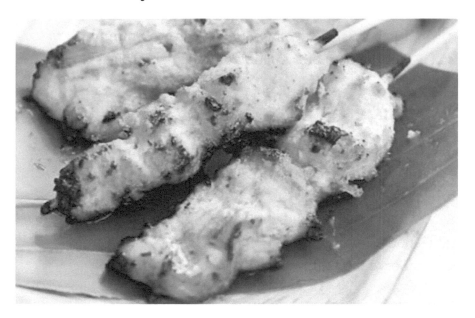

Ingredients:

- 4 skewers
- 1 teaspoon Splenda
- 1/4 teaspoon salt
- 1 tablespoon curry powder
- 1/2 cup light coconut milk
- Fresh ground black pepper, to taste
- 1 lb chicken breast, cut into strips
- Spray oil

How to prepare:

1. Soak wooden skewers in water overnight.
2. Blend coconut milk with pepper, curry powder, Splenda and salt in a bowl.

3.   Thread the chicken pieces on the skewers.

4.   Arrange the skewers on a baking sheet.

5.   Drizzle the marinade over the skewers and marinate for 30 minutes.

6.   Grill the skewers for 10 minutes on the medium-high heat while rotating constantly.

7.   Baste the skewers with the remaining marinade while grilling.

8.   Serve warm.

Preparation time: 5 minutes
Cooking time: 20 minutes
Total time: 25 minutes
Servings: 4

Nutritional Values:
- *Calories 152*
- *Total Fat 4 g*
- *Saturated Fat 2 g*
- *Cholesterol 65 mg*
- *Sodium 220 mg*
- *Total Carbs 2g*
- *Fiber 0 g*
- *Sugar 1 g*
- *Protein 26g*

Chicken Marsala

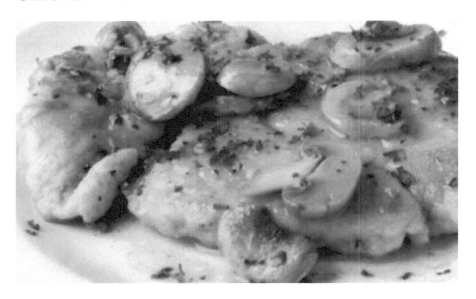

Ingredients:

- 2 (4 ounces) boneless skinless chicken breasts
- 3 tablespoon flour
- 1 teaspoon fresh ground black pepper
- 1 teaspoon dried oregano
- 1/2 cup mushrooms, sliced
- 1 teaspoon dried basil
- 1 tablespoon olive oil
- 1/4 cup marsala wine
- 1/2 teaspoon rice vinegar
- 1/4 teaspoon salt
- 1/4 cup low sodium vegetable stock

How to prepare:

1. Dice the chicken into 4 portions equally.

2.   Combine flour with oregano, basil, and pepper in a shallow bowl.

3.   Preheat olive oil in a large nonstick pan on high heat.

4.   Place the chicken in the flour mixture and dredge it to coat well.

5.   Sear the coated chicken in the pan for 3 minutes per side.

6.   Stir in mushrooms, salt, Marsala wine, and stock.

7.   Cook for 1 minute while mixing the sauce.

8.   Serve warm.

Preparation time: 10 minutes
Cooking time: 15 minutes

Total time: 25 minutes

Servings: 3

Nutritional Values:
- *Calories 188*
- *Total Fat 8 g*
- *Saturated Fat 1 g*
- *Cholesterol 0 mg*
- *Sodium 339 mg*
- *Total Carbs 8 g*
- *Fiber 1 g*
- *Sugar 2 g*
- *Protein 13g*

BEEF AND LAMB RECIPES

Pepper Steak

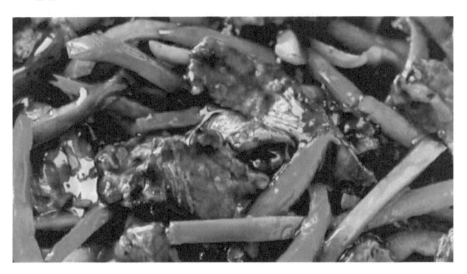

Ingredients:

*   3 tablespoons olive oil

*   2 lbs. beef sirloin, cut into strips

*   Garlic powder, to taste

*   1/4 cup beef broth

*   1 tablespoon xanthan gum

*   1/2 cup chopped onion

*   2 large green bell peppers, roughly chopped

*   1 red bell pepper, roughly chopped

*   3 tablespoons soy sauce

*   1 teaspoon Splenda

*   1 teaspoon salt

How to prepare:

1.   Season sirloin with garlic powder and set it aside.

2.   Hea oil in a pan and sear the beef until brown from both the sides.

3.   Transfer the beef to the slow cooker.

4.   Dissolve xanthan gum in some water and add to the cooker.

5.   Add all the remaining ingredients.

6.   Cover the dish with the lid then cook for 4 hours on high setting.

7.   Stir well and serve warm.

Preparation time: 10 minutes
Cooking time: 4 hours 10 minutes

Total time: 4 hours 20 minutes

Servings: 06

Nutritional Values:

- *Calories 301*
- *Total Fat 15.8 g*
- *Saturated Fat 2.7 g*
- *Cholesterol 75 mg*
- *Sodium 1189 mg*
- *Total Carbs 11.7 g*
- *Fibre 0.3g*
- *Sugar 0.1 g*
- *Protein 28.2 g*

Cuban Beef and Zucchini Kebabs

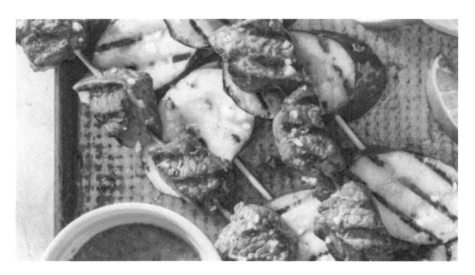

Ingredients:
- 1 (16 ounces) sirloin steak (1 inch thick), cut into 1 1/4-inch piece
- 8 (12-inch) wooden skewers
- 1/2 teaspoon salt
- 1/4 teaspoon black pepper
- 2 (10 ounces) zucchini, cut on a long diagonal into 1/2-inch-thick slices
- 2 tablespoons olive oil

How to prepare:
1. Heat the grill on medium high heat to 375 degrees F.
2. Thread beef on half of the skewers and season them with salt and pepper.

3. Thread zucchini slices on the remaining skewers and brush them with oil.

4. Place the skewers on the baking sheet.

5. Grill the 4 minutes per side while rotating constantly.

6. Grill the zucchini for 5 minutes per side.

7. Serve warm.

Preparation time: 10 minutes

Cooking time: 20 minutes

Total time: 30 minutes

Servings: 4

Nutritional Values:

- *Calories 308*
- *Total Fat 20.5 g*
- *Saturated Fat 3 g*
- *Cholesterol 0 mg*
- *Sodium 688 mg*
- *Total Carbs 10.3 g*
- *Sugar 1.4g*
- *Fiber 4.3 g*
- *Protein 49 g*

Flank Steak

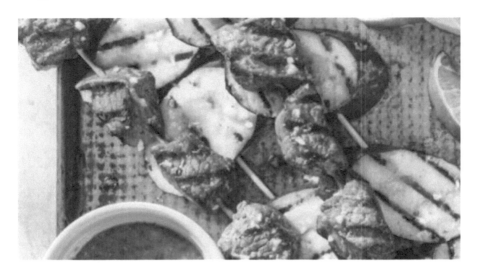

Ingredients:
- 1/4 cup honey
- 1/4 cup soy sauce
- 1/2 cup red wine
- 1 clove garlic, crushed
- 1 pinch dried rosemary, crushed
- 1 pinch hot chili powder (optional)
- 1 pinch freshly ground black pepper
- 1 pound flank steak

How to prepare:
1. Mix red wine, honey, soy sauce, rosemary, chili powder, pepper and garlic in a bowl.
2. Pour this marinade over the steak and let it marinate for 24 hours.

3. Preheat the grill over high heat and grease its grilling grate with oil.

4. Grill the steak for 7 mins per side.

5. Serve.

Preparation time: 10 minutes

Cooking time: 20 minutes

Total time: 30 minutes

Servings: 4

Nutritional Values:

- Calories 231
- Total Fat 20.1 g
- Saturated Fat 2.4 g
- Cholesterol 110 mg
- Sodium 941 mg
- Total Carbs 20.1 g
- Fiber 0.9 g
- Sugar 1.4 g
- Protein 14.6 g

Zucchini Meatloaf

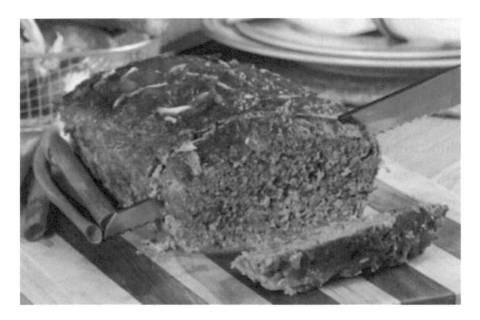

Ingredients:

- 1 tablespoon olive oil
- 1 green bell pepper, diced
- 1/2 cup diced sweet onion
- 1/2 teaspoon minced garlic
- 1 pound extra-lean (95%) ground beef
- 1 cup whole wheat bread crumbs
- 2 large egg whites
- 3/4 cup shredded carrot
- 3/4 cup shredded zucchini
- Salt and ground black pepper, to taste

How to prepare:

1.   Adjust the oven to 400 degrees F to preheat and grease a 9x5 inch loaf pan with oil.

2.   Preheat olive oil in a skillet and add onion and bell pepper.

3.   Saute for 10 minutes then add garlic. Stir cook for 2 minutes.

4.   Mix beef with egg whites, carrot, pepper, zucchini, salt, bell pepper and breadcrumbs in a bowl.

5.   Pour this mixture in the loaf pan and bake for 40 minutes.

6.   Slice and serve warm.

Preparation time: 10 minutes
Cooking time: 52 minutes
Total time: 62 minutes
Servings: 8

Nutritional Values:
- *Calories 280*
- *Total Fat 3.5 g*
- *Saturated Fat 0.1 g*
- *Cholesterol 320 mg*
- *Sodium 350 mg*
- *Total Carbs 7.6 g*
- *Fiber 0.7 g*
- *Sugar 0.7 g*
- *Protein 11.2 g*

Beef Picadillo

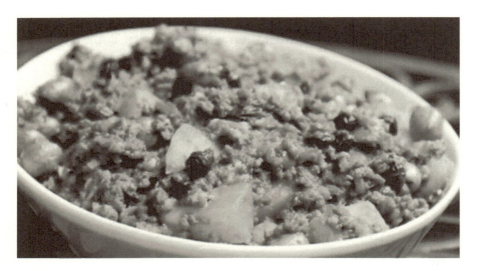

Ingredients:

- 2 pounds lean ground beef

- 1/4 cup olive oil

- 1/2 onion, chopped

- 1/2 green bell pepper, chopped

- 2 tablespoons minced garlic

- 2 (8 ounce) cans tomato sauce

- 2 cups water

- 1/2 cup red cooking wine

- 3 tablespoons hot sauce

- 1 (1.41 ounce) package sazon seasoning

- 1 tablespoon chopped fresh parsley

- 1/2 teaspoon garlic powder

- 1/2 teaspoon onion powder

- 1/2 teaspoon ground cumin

- 1/2 teaspoon ground black pepper

- 1/4 teaspoon ground bay leaf

- 3 ounces Spanish-style olives

- 1 teaspoon salt, or to taste

- 1 small almond butternut squash, peeled and cut into cubes

How to prepare:

1. Saute ground beef in a greased skillet for 10 minutes until al dente.

2. Transfer beef to a plate.

3. Preheat olive oil in a nonstick pan then add pepper, garlic, and onion.

4. Saute for 3 minutes then stir in beef.

5. Add wine, water, hot sauce, parsley, garlic powder, sazon seasoning, cumin, pepper, bay leaf, and onion powder.

6. Cook on low simmer for 10 minutes.

7. Add squash and olives. Cook for another 45 minutes.

8. Adjust seasoning with salt.

9. Serve warm.

Preparation time: 10 minutes

Cooking time: 1 hour 15 minutes

Total time: 1 hour 25 minutes

Servings: 8

Nutritional Values:

- *Calories 472*
- *Total Fat 11.1 g*
- *Saturated Fat 5.8 g*
- *Cholesterol 610 mg*
- *Sodium 749 mg*
- *Total Carbs 19.9 g*
- *Fiber 0.2 g*
- *Sugar 0.2 g*
- *Protein 13.5 g*

Lamb Tagine

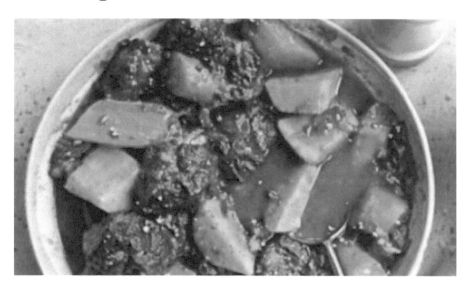

Ingredients:

- 1 onion, finely chopped
- 1 tablespoon ground cumin
- 2 teaspoons ground cinnamon
- 1 teaspoon turmeric
- 2 teaspoons coriander
- 1 teaspoon dried red chili flakes
- 1 lb. lean lamb leg steaks, cut into bite-sized pieces
- 1 cup fat-free yogurt
- 2 teaspoons Splenda
- 4 carrots, cut into large pieces
- 2 courgettes, sliced
- Fresh coriander, to garnish

How to prepare:

1. Add onion, lamb, and spices to a greased pan then saute for 6 minutes.

2. Stir in sweetener and yogurt.

3. Boil the mixture then reduce the heat.

4. Cover the pot with the lid then cook for 35 minutes until meat is al dente.

5. Add courgettes and carrots.

6. Cook for 15 minutes.

7. Garnish with coriander.

8. Serve.

Preparation time: 5 minutes
Cooking time: 55 minutes

Total time: 60 minutes

Servings: 4

Nutritional Values:

*   Calories 327
*   Total Fat 3.5 g
*   Saturated Fat 0.5 g
*   Cholesterol 162 mg
*   Sodium 142 mg
*   Total Carbs 33.6g
*   Fiber 0.4 g
*   Sugar 0.5 g
*   Protein 24.5 g

Grilled lamb & potato crush

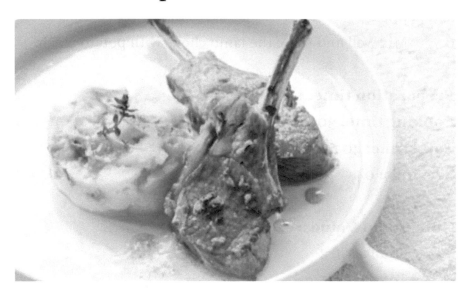

Ingredients:

- 1 lb. bag new potato
- Zest 1 lemon
- 1 tablespoon olive oil
- 4 lamb chops or steaks
- 1 garlic clove, crushed
- ½ lb. bag baby spinach

How to prepare:

1. Preheat the grill to high.
2. Season the lamb chops with oil, lemon zest, salt, and pepper.
3. Grill the chops for 10 minutes until golden brown.
4. Boil potatoes in water for 20 minutes then drain them.

5. Mash the boiled potatoes and mix with spinach, salt, and pepper.

6. Mix well and serve the lamb chops with potato mash.

Preparation time: 10 minutes

Cooking time: 30 minutes

Total time: 40 minutes

Servings: 04

Nutritional Values:

- *Calories 413*
- *Total Fat 7.5 g*
- *Saturated Fat 1.1 g*
- *Cholesterol 20 mg*
- *Sodium 97 mg*
- *Total Carbs 41.4 g*
- *Fiber 0 g*
- *Sugar 0 g*
- *Protein 21.1g*

Chilli Ginger Lamb Chops

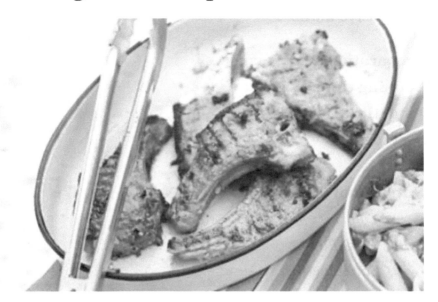

Ingredients:

- 4 garlic cloves, crushed
- 1 tablespoon grated ginger
- 2 tablespoon olive oil
- ½ teaspoon chili powder
- 1 teaspoon cumin
- 8 lamb chops

How to prepare:

1.	Mix garlic with ginger, spices, seasoning, and oil in a blender.

2.	Season the lamb chops with this spice mixture and refrigerate overnight.

3.	Preheat a grill over medium heat.

4. Grill the chops for 3 mins per side.

5. Serve warm.

Preparation time: 5 minutes

Cooking time: 12 minutes

Total time: 17 minutes

Servings: 08

Nutritional Values:

- *Calories 253*
- *Total Fat 7.5 g*
- *Saturated Fat 1.1 g*
- *Cholesterol 20 mg*
- *Sodium 297 mg*
- *Total Carbs 10.4 g*
- *Fiber 0 g*
- *Sugar 0 g*
- *Protein 13.1g*

Lamb Dopiaza

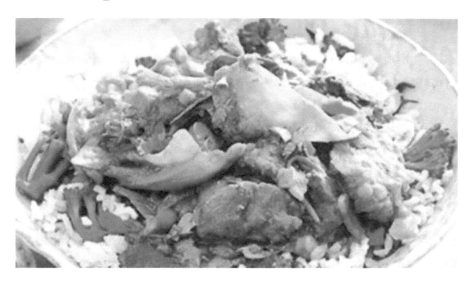

Ingredients:
- ½ lb. lamb leg steaks, cut into 2? cm/ 1in chunks
- 1 cup yogurt, plus 4 tablespoons to serve
- 1 tablespoon medium curry powder
- 2 teaspoons cold-pressed rapeseed oil
- 2 medium onions, 1 thinly sliced, 1 cut into 5 wedges
- 2 garlic cloves, peeled and finely sliced
- 1 tablespoon ginger, peeled and finely chopped
- 1 small red chili, finely chopped
- ¼ cup dried split red lentils, rinsed
- ½ small pack of coriander, roughly chopped, plus extra to garnish
- 1 cup pack baby leaf spinach

How to prepare:
1.   Season the lamb with black pepper, ? tablespoon curry powder and yogurt.

2.   Preheat half of the oil in a pan. Add onion wedges and saute for 5 minutes.

3.   Transfer the wedges to a plate.

4.   Pour remaining oil into the same pan then add garlic, ginger, chili, and sliced onion.

5.   Saute for 3 minutes then decrease the heat.

6.   Add remaining powder. Cook for 1 minute.

7.   Mix well and cook for 5 minutes on medium-high heat.

8.   Pour in water along with coriander and lentils.

9.   Cover the dish with the lid then cook for 45 minutes on low heat.

10.   Uncover and stir well. Cook for 15 minutes on low heat.

11.   Stir in onion wedges and cook for 15 minutes.

12.   Add spinach leaves. Let it rest for 5 minutes.

13.   Serve warm with brown rice.

Preparation time: 5 minutes
Cooking time: 1 hour 30 minutes
Total time: 1 hour 35 minutes
Servings: 04

Nutritional Values:

- *Calories 201*
- *Total Fat 5.5 g*
- *Saturated Fat 2.1 g*
- *Cholesterol 10 mg*
- *Sodium 597 mg*
- *Total Carbs 2.4 g*
- *Fiber 0 g*
- *Sugar 0 g*
- *Protein 3.1g*

Mediterranean Vegetables with Lamb

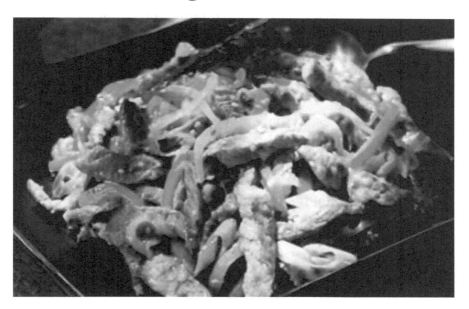

Ingredients:
- 1 tablespoon olive oil
- ½ lb. lean lamb fillet, thinly sliced
- 2 shallots, halved
- 2 large courgettes, cut into chunks
- ½ teaspoon ground cumin,
- ½ teaspoon paprika
- ½ teaspoon coriander, ground
- 1 red, 1 green pepper, and 1 orange pepper cut into squares
- 1 garlic clove, sliced
- 2 cups vegetable stock
- A handful of coriander leaves, roughly chopped

How to prepare:

1.   Heat a greased pan and add lamb and shallots to the pan.

2.   Saute for 3 minutes then stir in courgettes. Cook for 4 minutes.

3.   Stir in spices, garlic, and peppers. Decrease the heat and cook for 5 minutes.

4.   Add in stock and seasoning.

5.   Cover and let it simmer for 15 minutes.

6.   Garnish with coriander and serve warm.

Preparation time: 10 minutes

Cooking time: 30 minutes

Total time: 40 minutes

Servings: 04

Nutritional Values:

- *Calories 413*
- *Total Fat 8.5 g*
- *Saturated Fat 3.1 g*
- *Cholesterol 120 mg*
- *Sodium 497 mg*
- *Total Carbs 21.4 g*
- *Fiber 0.6 g*
- *Sugar 0.1 g*
- *Protein 14.1g*

SNACK AND SWEETS RECIPES

Blueberry Cherry Crisp

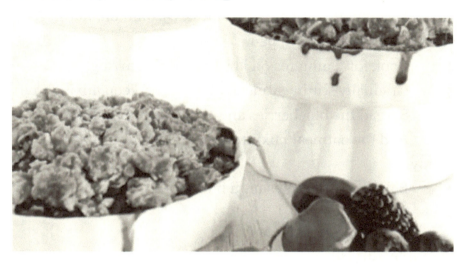

Ingredients:
- 1 cup old-fashioned oatmeal
- 1/3 cup coconut flour
- 1/2 cup chopped macadamia nuts
- 2 tablespoons coconut oil
- 3 tablespoons almond butter
- 2 tablespoons honey
- 1 teaspoon cinnamon
- 1/4 teaspoon nutmeg
- 1/8 teaspoon sea salt
- 4 cups frozen cherries, thawed
- 2 cups frozen blueberries

How to prepare:

1.   Set the oven to 375 degrees F. Almond butter a 9x9 inch glass dish.

2.   Mix oatmeal with nuts and flours in a glass bowl.

3.   Heat honey with almond butter, coconut oil, nutmeg, sea salt and cinnamon in pan.

4.   Cook for 3 minutes on low heat while stirring.

5.   Gradually stir in oatmeal mixture and keep mixing well.

6.   Spread the blueberries and cherries in the glass dish.

7.   Add the oatmeal mixture to the dish and spread it evenly.

8.   Bake for 35 minutes until bubbly.

9.   Serve,

Preparation time: 5 minutes
Cooking time: 35 minutes

Total time: 45 minutes

Servings: 8

Nutritional Values:

- *Calories 252*
- *Total Fat 16 g*
- *Saturated Fat 7 g*
- *Cholesterol 11 mg*
- *Sodium 8 mg*
- *Total Carbs 29 g*
- *Sugar 1.8 g*
- *Fiber 5 g*
- *Protein 4 g*

Baked Apples with Tahini Raisin Filling

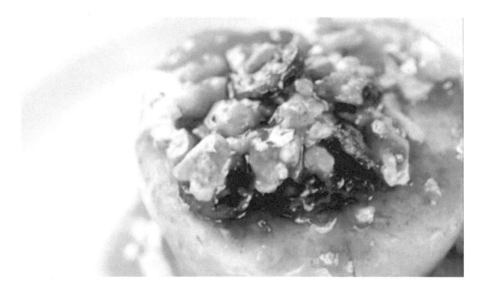

Ingredients:

- 4 ripe apples, cored

- 3/4 cup tahini

- 1 cup apple juice

- 3 tablespoons raisins

- 1/3 cup chopped pecans

- 1/4 teaspoon cinnamon

- Dash of nutmeg

- Dash of vanilla

- 3/4 cup boiling water

How to prepare:

1. Set the oven to 375 degrees F to preheat. Grease a 9x13-inch baking dish with oil.

2. Place the cored apples in the shallow dish.

3.   Mix tahini with half cup apple juice in a small bowl.

4.   Stir in pecans, raisins, nutmeg, vanilla, and cinnamon. Mix well.

5.   Stuff this mixture into the core of the apples.

6.   Add some boiling water to the baking dish.

7.   Pour the remaining apple juice on top.

8.   Bake for 35 minutes until tender.

9.   Serve the apples with the remaining juices on top.

Preparation time: 10 minutes

Cooking time: 35 minutes

Total time: 45 minutes

Servings: 4

Nutritional Values:
- *Calories 386*
- *Total Fat 24 g*
- *Saturated Fat 3 g*
- *Cholesterol 0 mg*
- *Sodium 19 mg*
- *Total Carbs 41 g*
- *Sugar 1.9 g*
- *Fiber 7 g*
- *Protein 8 g*

Coconut Rice Pudding

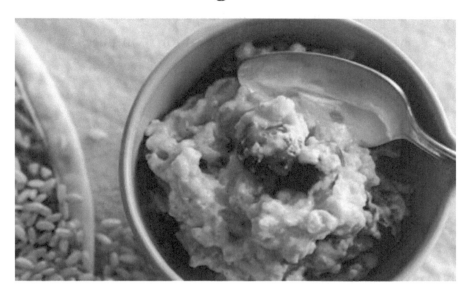

Ingredients:

- 3/4 cup low-fat milk
- 1/2 cup coconut milk
- 1 large pear grated
- 2 tablespoons honey
- ¼ cup dried cranberries
- 1 (1oz) package fat-free, sugar-free vanilla pudding mix
- 2 cups cooked brown rice
- 1/4 cup shredded coconut
- 1/2 teaspoon ground ginger

How to prepare:

1.   Cook grates pears with milk, coconut milk, and honey in a pan on medium heat.

2. Boil the mixture then remove it from the heat.

3. Gradually stir in pudding mix, coconut, ginger, and rice.

4. Mix well and let this mixture sit for 10 minutes.

5. Stir in cranberries and mix gently.

6. Serve.

Preparation time: 5 minutes

Cooking time: 10 minutes

Total time: 15 minutes

Servings: 4

Nutritional Values:

- *Calories 190*
- *Total Fat 6 g*
- *Saturated Fat 2 g*
- *Cholesterol 2 mg*
- *Sodium 244 mg*
- *Total Carbs 31 g*
- *Sugar 3.6 g*
- *Fiber 0.8 g*
- *Protein 3 g*

Peach Cobbler

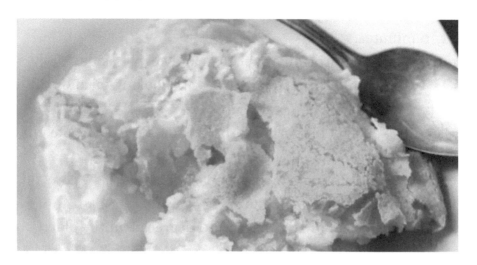

Ingredients:
- 1/2 teaspoon ground cinnamon
- 1 tablespoon vanilla extract
- 2 tablespoons xanthan gum
- 1/4 cup peach juice
- 1 cup peach nectar
- 1-3/4 lbs. fresh peaches, sliced
- 1 tablespoon margarine
- 1 cup dry pancake mix
- 2/3 cup coconut flour
- 1/2 cup Splenda
- 2/3 cup evaporated skim milk

Topping: 1/2 teaspoon nutmeg and 1 tablespoon Splenda

How to prepare:
1.   Whisk vanilla with peach, nectar, peach juice, xanthan gum and cinnamon in a pan.

2. Cook well until it bubbles and thickens.

3. Stir in sliced peaches and reduce the heat. Let it simmer for 10 minutes.

4. Heat margarine in a saucepan and keep it aside.

5. Grease an 8-inch square dish with cooking oil and add the peach mixture.

6. Mix melted margarine with Splenda, flour, pancake mix and milk in a separate bowl.

7. Pour this mixture over the peach mixture.

8. Sprinkle Splenda and nutmeg over it.

9. Bake for about 20 mins at 400 degrees F until golden brown.

10. Slice and serve.

Preparation time: 10 minutes
Cooking time: 30 minutes
Total time: 40 minutes
Servings: 6

Nutritional Values:
- *Calories 271*
- *Total Fat 4 g*
- *Saturated Fat 1 g*
- *Cholesterol 0 mg*
- *Sodium 263 mg*
- *Total Carbs 9.6 g*
- *Sugar 0.1 g*
- *Fiber 3.8 g*
- *Protein 7.6 g*

Vanilla parfait Vanilla parfait

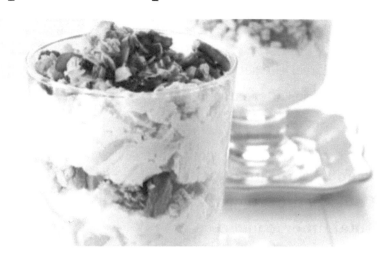

Ingredients:

- 1 cup vanilla milk (unsweetened)
- 1 cup greek yogurt (plain low fat)
- 2 tablespoon agave
- 1 teaspoon vanilla
- 1/8 teaspoon kosher salt
- 1/4 cup chia seeds
- 2 cups sliced strawberries
- 1/4 cup sliced almonds
- 4 teaspoon agave for serving

How to prepare:

1.   Mix milk, yogurt, agave, vanilla, and salt in a medium bowl.

2.   Whisk in chia seeds and let it rest for 25 minutes.

3.   Cover the bowl and refrigerate it overnight.

4.   Mix strawberries with agave and toasted almonds in a bowl.

5.   Layer the serving glasses with yogurt pudding and strawberries alternatively.

6.   Serve.

Preparation time: 10 minutes

Cooking time: 0 minutes

Total time: 10 minutes

Servings: 2

Nutritional Values:

- *Calories 199*
- *Total Fat 7g*
- *Saturated Fat 3.5 g*
- *Cholesterol 125 mg*
- *Total Carbs 7.2 g*
- *Sugar 1.4 g*
- *Fiber 2.1 g*
- *Sodium 135 mg*
- *Protein 4.7 g*

Pumpkin Pudding Parfaits

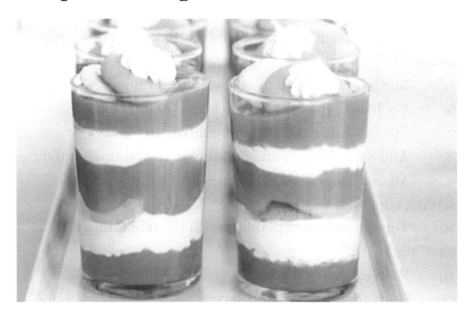

Ingredients:

- 1 cup pumpkin puree
- 1/4 cup packed Splenda
- 1/2 teaspoon ground cinnamon
- 3 cup almond milk
- 2 tablespoons almond butter
- 1/2 cup Splenda
- 3 tablespoons xanthan gum
- 1 teaspoon salt
- 4 large egg whites
- 2 teaspoon vanilla extract

How to prepare:

1.   Mix pumpkin puree with cinnamon, and Splenda in a saucepan.

2.   Stir cook the mixture for 10 minutes until smooth.

3.　　Heat 2 cups of milk with almond butter in a microwave for 2 minutes on high heat.

4.　　Whisk Splenda with salt and xanthan gum in a large pan.

5.　　Stir in 1 cup milk and mix well until smooth.

6.　　Cook until the mixture thickens.

7.　　Stir in vanilla and strain the mixture.

8.　　Add half of the vanilla pudding to the pumpkin mixture.

9.　　Mix well and divide the pumpkin pudding into the serving cups.

10.　　Top the pumpkin pudding with the remaining vanilla pudding.

11.　　Refrigerate for 4 hours.

12.　　Garnish as desired and serve.

Preparation time: 10 minutes
Cooking time: 22 minutes
Total time: 32 minutes
Servings: 6

Nutritional Values:
- Calories 151
- Total Fat 3.4 g
- Saturated Fat 7 g
- Cholesterol 20 mg
- Total Carbs 6.4 g
- Sugar 2.1 g
- Fiber 4.8 g
- Sodium 136 mg
- Protein 4.2 g

Banana Pudding Parfaits

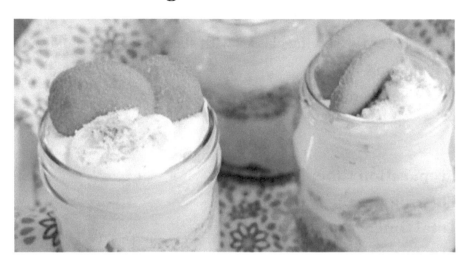

Ingredients:

- 1 cup Splenda
- 1/4 cup xanthan gum
- 1/4 teaspoon salt
- 2 1/2 cups almond milk
- 4 large egg whites
- 2 tablespoons unsalted almond butter
- 1 teaspoon pure vanilla extract
- 2 bananas, sliced
- 12 shortbread cookies, crumbled

How to prepare:

1. Mix Splenda with salt, xanthan gum, and milk in a saucepan.

2. Stir cook until smooth then whisk in egg whites.

3. Cook until the mixture bubbles.

4. Strain the mixture and stir in vanilla and almond butter. Mix well.

5. Layer the serving glasses with slices bananas, cookies, and pudding.

6. Refrigerate for 1 hour.

7. Serve.

Preparation time: 10 minutes

Cooking time: 15minutes

Total time: 25 minutes

Servings: 2

Nutritional Values:

- *Calories 165*
- *Total Fat 3 g*
- *Saturated Fat 0.2 g*
- *Cholesterol 09 mg*
- *Sodium 7.1 mg*
- *Total Carbs 17.5 g*
- *Sugar 1.1 g*
- *Fiber 0.5 g*
- *Protein 2.2 g*

Oatmeal Cookies

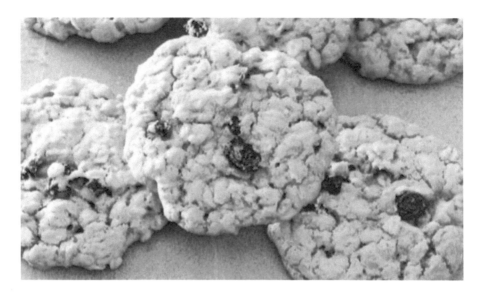

Ingredients:

- 1 cup coconut flour

- 1 cup quick-cooking oats

- 1/2 cup Splenda

- 1/2 teaspoon baking powder

- 1/2 teaspoon baking soda

- 1/2 teaspoon salt

- 1/2 teaspoon ground cinnamon

- 2 egg whites

- 1/3 cup corn syrup

- 1 teaspoon vanilla extract

- 1/3 cup raisins

How to prepare:

1.   Mix flour with oats, baking powder, soda, salt, cinnamon and Splenda in a bowl.

2.   Fold in raisins and mix gently.

3.   Drop the batter on the baking sheet spoon by spoon.

4.   Bake at 375 degrees F in the preheated oven for 10 mins.

5.   Serve.

Preparation time: 5 minutes

Cooking time: 10 minutes

Total time: 15 minutes

Servings: 6

Nutritional Values:

- *Calories 102*
- *Total Fat 1 g*
- *Saturated Fat 0 g*
- *Cholesterol 0 mg*
- *Sodium 138 mg*
- *Total Carbs 24 g*
- *Fibre 0g*
- *Sugar 0 g*
- *Protein 2 g*

Gingersnaps Gingersnaps

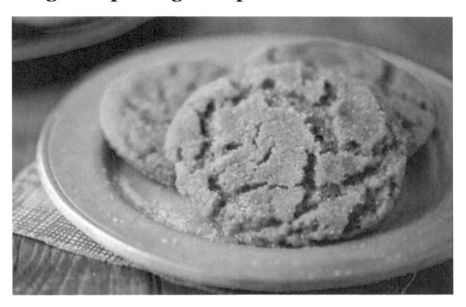

Ingredients:
- 1/2 cup unsulphured molasses
- 1 egg white
- 3 1/2 cups coconut flour
- 1 teaspoon baking soda
- 1/2 teaspoon salt
- 2 teaspoons ground ginger
- 1 teaspoon cinnamon
- 1/2 teaspoon ground cloves
- 1/2 teaspoon ground nutmeg
- 1/2 teaspoon freshly ground black pepper

How to prepare:
1. Whisk almond butter with Splenda in a bowl.
2. Stir in molasses and egg white. Mix well until smooth.

3. Combine flour with salt, spices, and baking soda in a mixing bowl.

4. Stir in almond butter mixture and mix well on low speed.

5. Divide the dough into two halves. Wrap the dough in a plastic sheet.

6. Refrigerate it for 3 hours.

7. Set the oven to 350 degrees F.

8. Unwrap the dough and keep it on a floured surface.

9. Roll the dough into 1/8 inch thick sheet.

10. Cut small cookies using a cookie cutter.

11. Set the cookies on a baking sheet lined with parchment paper.

12. Bake for 8 minutes until golden brown.

13. Serve.

Preparation time: 10 minutes
Cooking time: 8 minutes
Total time: 18 minutes
Servings: 6

Nutritional Values:
- Calories 209
- Total Fat 0.5 g
- Saturated Fat 11.7 g
- Cholesterol 58 mg
- Sodium 163 mg
- Total Carbs 19.9 g
- Fiber 1.5 g
- Sugar 0.3 g
- Protein 3.3 g

Coconut Biscotti

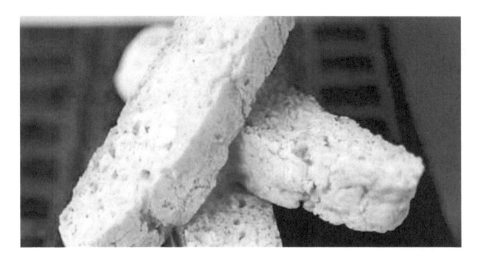

Ingredients:
- 1 1/2 cups coconut flour
- 3/4 teaspoon baking powder
- 1/4 teaspoon salt
- 1/4 teaspoon baking soda
- 1/8 teaspoon grated whole nutmeg
- 3/4 cup Splenda
- 1 teaspoon vanilla extract
- 2 egg whites
- 1 cup flaked sweetened coconut

How to prepare:
1. Set the oven to 300 degrees F to preheat.
2. Mix all the ingredients in an electric mixer to form a smooth dough.

3.   Knead the dough then make 3-inch rolls out of this dough.

4.   Place the rolls on the baking sheet lined with parchment paper.

5.   Lightly press each roll and bake for 40 minutes at 300 degrees F.

6.   Allow them to cool then diagonally slice the rolls.

7.   Bake for another 20 minutes.

8.   Serve.

Preparation time: 10 minutes

Cooking time: 60 minutes

Total time: 1 hour 10 minutes

Servings: 6

Nutritional Values:

- *Calories 237*
- *Total Fat 19.8 g*
- *Saturated Fat 1.4 g*
- *Cholesterol 10 mg*
- *Sodium 719 mg*
- *Total Carbs 55.1 g*
- *Fiber 0.9 g*
- *Sugar 1.4 g*
- *Protein 17.8 g*

SAUCES AND CONDIMENTS RECIPES

Light Romesco Sauce

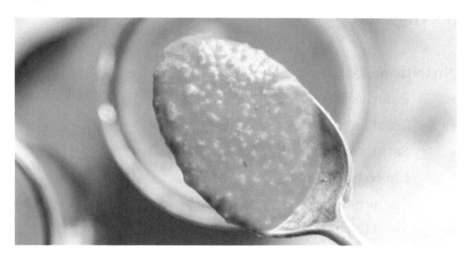

Ingredients:

- 1/2 cup canned artichoke hearts, drained
- 1 piece jarred roasted piquillo or red pepper
- 4 tablespoon vegetable or chicken broth
- 2 teaspoon olive oil
- 1/8 teaspoon dried thyme
- 1/8 teaspoon onion powder
- A handful of fresh chopped herbs
- Sea salt, to taste

How to prepare:

1. Blend everything in a blend until smooth.
2. Serve and use as desired.

Preparation time: 5 minutes

Cooking time: 0 minutes

Total time: 5 minutes

Servings: 12

Nutritional Values:

- Calories 86
- Total Fat 0.9 g
- Saturated Fat 8.1 g
- Cholesterol 0 mg
- Sodium 8 mg
- Total Carbs 8.3 g
- Sugar 1.8 g
- Fiber 3.8 g
- Protein 1.4 g

Creamy Cauliflower Alfredo

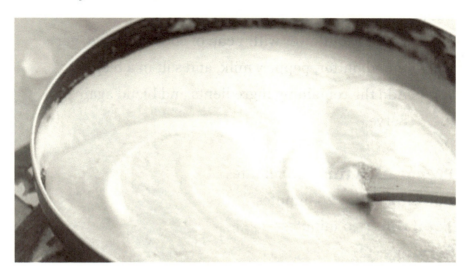

Ingredients:

- 8 large cloves garlic, minced
- 2 tablespoons almond butter
- 6 cups cauliflower florets
- 7 cups vegetable broth or water
- 1 teaspoon salt
- ½ teaspoon pepper
- ½ cup almond milk

How to prepare:

1. Melt almond butter in a pan and add garlic to saute until golden brown.
2. Set the garlic aside.
3. Heat broth in a large pot over high heat.
4. Stir in cauliflower florets and cook for 10 minutes.

5.   Drain the cauliflower and reserve 2 cups of the cooking liquid.

6.   Blend cauliflower with 1 cup of cooking liquid, garlic with almond butter, pepper, milk, and salt in a blender.

7.   Add the remaining ingredients and blend again.

8.   Serve.

Preparation time: 10 minutes

Cooking time: 20 minutes

Total time: 30 minutes

Servings: 12

Nutritional Values:

- Calories 58
- Total Fat 3 g
- Saturated Fat 0.8 g
- Cholesterol 5 mg
- Sodium 123 mg
- Total Carbs 6 g
- Sugar 1.9 g
- Fiber 2.1 g
- Protein 2 g

Arugula Pesto

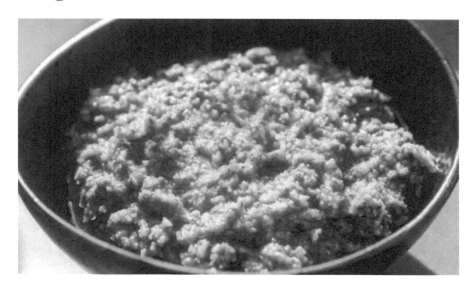

Ingredients:
- 2 tablespoon pine nuts

- 2 cloves garlic, minced

- 4 cups fresh arugula

- 2 tablespoon water

- 2 teaspoon stevia

- 1/4 teaspoon salt

- 1 tablespoon rice vinegar

- 2 tablespoons olive oil

How to prepare:

1. Blend all the ingredients in a blender.

2. Serve.

Preparation time: 5 minutes

Cooking time: 0 minutes

Total time: 5 minutes

Servings: 12

Nutritional Values:

- Calories 83
- Total Fat 8 g
- Saturated Fat 2 g
- Cholesterol 1 mg
- Sodium 43 mg
- Total Carbs 1 g
- Sugar 0 g
- Fiber 0 g
- Protein 3 g

Thai Peanut Sauce

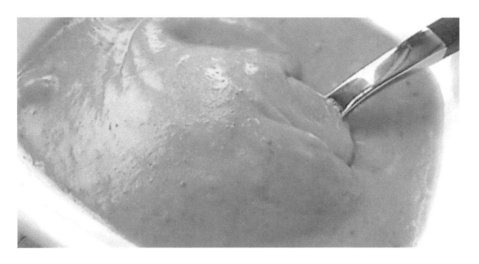

Ingredients:

- 1/4 cup reduced-fat peanut almond butter
- 6 tablespoon vegetable broth
- 1/4 cup coconut milk
- 2 teaspoons low-sodium soy sauce
- 2 teaspoons rice vinegar
- 2 teaspoons Tabasco sauce

How to prepare:

1. Blend everything a food processor.
2. Serve.

Preparation time: 5 minutes

Cooking time: 0 minutes

Total time: 5 minutes

Servings: 8

Nutritional Values:

- Calories 45
- Total Fat 3 g
- Saturated Fat 1 g
- Cholesterol 0 mg
- Total Carbs 3 g
- Sodium 93 mg
- Sugar 1 g
- Fiber 0 g
- Protein 2 g

Pumpkin Alfredo sauce

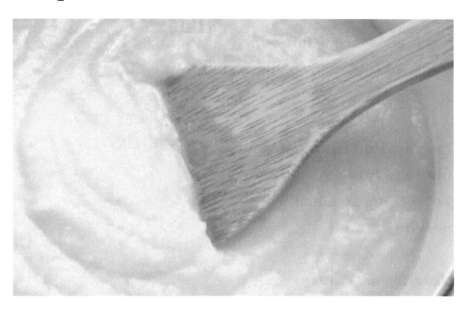

Ingredients:

- 3 cloves garlic, minced
- 1 stick (1/2 cup) unsalted almond butter
- 4 ounces coconut cream
- 3/4 cup pumpkin puree
- 1/2 cup almond milk
- 1 tablespoon xanthan gum
- 1 teaspoon Italian seasoning
- Salt and pepper, to taste

How to prepare:

1. Saute garlic in a saucepan on medium heat.
2. Stir in almond butter, pumpkin, and coconut cream.
3. Mix well and cook on low heat.

4.   Whisk xanthan gum with milk and add this slurry to the sauce.

5.   Cook the mixture until it thickens.

6.   Add seasoning to the mixture. Mix well.

7.   Serve.

Preparation time: 5 minutes

Cooking time: 15 minutes

Total time: 20 minutes

Servings: 12

Nutritional Values:

- *Calories 92*
- *Total Fat 7.4 g*
- *Saturated Fat 1.5 g*
- *Cholesterol 125 mg*
- *Sodium 135 mg*
- *Total Carbs 2.2 g*
- *Sugar 1.4 g*
- *Fiber 2.1 g*
- *Protein 4.7 g*

Apple Almond Butter

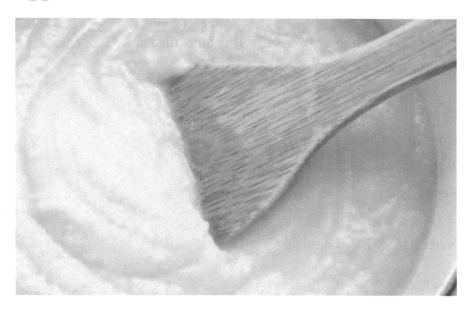

Ingredients:

- 4 cups Splenda
- 3 teaspoons ground cinnamon
- 1/4 teaspoon ground cloves
- 1/4 teaspoon salt

How to prepare:

1. Add apples, cinnamon, salt, Splenda, and cloves to a slow cooker.

2. Cover the cooker and let it cook for 1 hour on high settings.

3. Decrease the heat to low and cook for 11 hours until the mixture darkens.

4.   Remove the lid of the cooker then cook for another hour.

5.   Blend the mixture until it is smooth.

6.   Serve or store for later use.

Preparation time: 5 minutes

Cooking time: 12 hours

Total time: 12 hours 5 minutes

Servings: 12

Nutritional Values:

- *Calories 68*
- *Total Fat 0 g*
- *Saturated 0 g*
- *Cholesterol 0 mg*
- *Sodium 9 mg*
- *Total Carbs 17 g*
- *Sugar 16 g*
- *Fiber 1 g*
- *Protein 0 g*

Honey Mustard

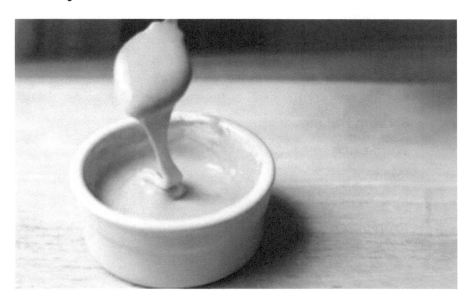

Ingredients:

- 1/2 cup stone-ground mustard

- 1/4 cup honey

- 1/4 cup rice vinegar

How to prepare:

1. Mix everything in a glass bowl.

2. Serve or store for later use.

Preparation time: 5 minutes

Cooking time: 0 minutes

Total time: 5 minutes

Servings: 12

Nutritional Values:

- *Calories 28*
- *Total Fat 1 g*
- *Saturated Fat 0 g*
- *Cholesterol 0 mg*
- *Sodium 154 mg*
- *Total Carbs 6 g*
- *Sugar 5 g*
- *Fiber 0 g*
- *Protein 0 g*

Avocado Sauce

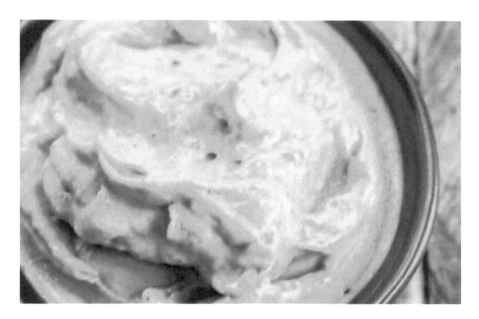

Ingredients:
- 1 ripe avocado

- 1/2 teaspoon salt

- 1 jalapeno, stemmed, cut into pieces

- 2 tablespoons chopped cilantro

- 1/2 cup cold water

- 2 teaspoons olive oil

- 1 tablespoon roughly chopped onion

How to prepare:
1. Blend everything in a blender until smooth.

2. Serve.

Preparation time: 5 minutes
Cooking time: 0 minutes

Total time: 5 minutes

Servings: 6

Nutritional Values:

- *Calories 3*
- *Total Fat 0 g*
- *Saturated Fat 0 g*
- *Cholesterol 0 mg*
- *Sodium 30 mg*
- *Total Carbs 1g*
- *Fibre 0g*
- *Sugar 0 g*
- *Protein 0 g*

Spiced Maple Mustard

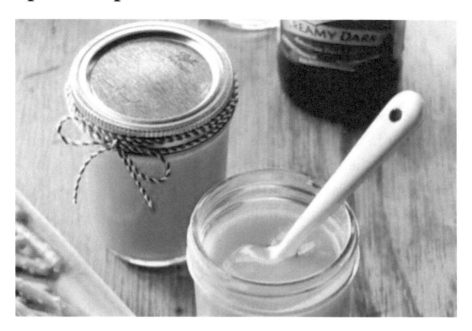

Ingredients:

- 1 teaspoon whole allspice
- 1 cup water, divided
- 1/2 cup rice vinegar
- 1/4 cup maple syrup
- 1 tablespoon coconut flour
- 1 tablespoon xanthan gum
- 2 teaspoons ground mustard
- 1 teaspoon ground turmeric
- 3/4 teaspoon salt

How to prepare:

1.   Tie all spices in a cheesecloth tightly.

2.   Mix ? cup water, maple syrup, and vinegar in a saucepan then set it aside.

3.   Mix mustard, turmeric, xanthan gum, flour, remaining water and salt in a pan.

4.   Stir in the maple syrup mixture gradually.

5.   Place the spice bag in the pan and let it simmer for 10 minutes with occasional stirring.

6.   Remove and discard the spice bag.

7.   Allow it to cool.

8.   Serve or store in the refrigerator.

Preparation time: 10 minutes
Cooking time: 0 minutes

Total time: 10 minutes

Servings: 2

Nutritional Values:
* *Calories 19*
* *Total Fat 0 g*
* *Saturated Fat 0 g*
* *Cholesterol 0 mg*
* *Sodium 111 mg*
* *Total Carbs 4 g*
* *Fiber 0 g*
* *Sugar 3 g*
* *Protein 0 g*

Apple Cranberry Sauce

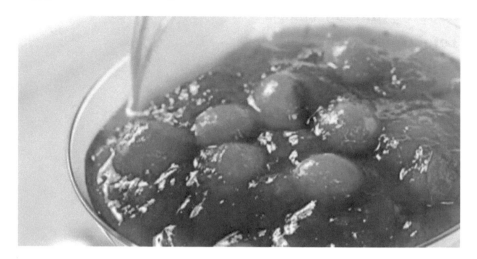

Ingredients:
- 1 cup fresh or frozen cranberries
- 6 large apples, peeled and coarsely chopped
- 1/2 cup Splenda
- 1/3 cup apple juice
- 1/4 teaspoon ground mace
- 1/8 teaspoon ground coriander

How to prepare:
1. Mix and boil the all the ingredients in a saucepan.
2. Decrease the heat and let it simmer for 15 minutes.
3. Puree the sauce using a handheld blender.
4. Cover the sauce and refrigerate.
5. Use a desired.

Preparation time: 5 minutes

Cooking time: 15 minutes

Total time: 20 minutes

Servings: 12

Nutritional Values:

- *Calories 124*
- *Total Fat 0 g*
- *Saturated Fat 0 g*
- *Cholesterol 0 mg*
- *Sodium 1 mg*
- *Total Carbs 32g*
- *Fiber 2 g*
- *Sugar 28 g*
- *Protein 0 g*

Conclusion

The modern day diet we are consuming is way more acidic than it previously was. This imbalanced acid alkali diet is the reason for very serious and chronic medical complications like arthritis and osteoporosis etc. Creating a balanced acid alkali diet plan is very critical for having access to a healthy lifestyle, and it is very easy to achieve. Apart from weight loss, the alkaline diet is high in energy, lowers the risk of having kidney complications, type-2 diabetes, and various other diseases.

A combination of lean proteins, comparatively slow low-carbs, and fats can prove to be very pivotal to lose weight which indeed helps in lowering the risk of having GERD in the first place. Beginners should go for a protein shake in breakfast for having an effective and faster approach towards weight loss.

Alkaline foods like legumes, fruits, roots, nuts, and veggies should be consumed in abundance. Opt for these foods rather than meats and grains. Go for green or dark veggies like avocados, beetroot, kale, spinach, etc. It's not necessary to completely boycott meats, refined sugars, dairy, and grains but it is preferred to lower their intake to lower down the acidity of your body.